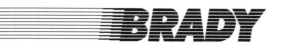

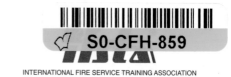

INTERNATIONAL FIRE SERVICE TRAINING ASSOCIATION

EMERGENCY INCIDENT REHABILITATION

EDWARD T. DICKINSON
MD, NREMT-P, FACEP

MICHAEL A. WIEDER
MS, CFPS

Brady/Prentice Hall
Upper Saddle River, New Jersey 07458

Library of Congress Cataloging-in-Publication Data

Dickinson, Edward T.
    Emergency incident rehabilitation / Edward T. Dickinson, Michael A. Wieder.
      p. cm.
    Includes bibliographical references and index.
    ISBN 0-8359-5375-0
      1. Fire fighters—Health and hygiene.   2. Emergency medical personnel—Health and
hygiene.   3. Fire fighters—Rehabilitation.   4. Emergency medical personnel—
Rehabilitation.   I. Wieder, Michael A.   II. Title.
    RC965.F48D53   2000
    628.9'25'0289—dc21   99-39052
                                                                            CIP

Publisher: Julie Alexander
Managing Development Editor: Lois Berlowitz
Project Editor: Dan Zinkus
Marketing Manager: Tiffany Price
Manufacturing Manager: Ilene Sanford
Managing Production Editor: Patrick Walsh
Production Liaison: Larry Hayden
Art Director: Marianne Frasco
Full Service Production/Composition: BookMasters, Inc.
Cover Printer: Phoenix Color
Printer/Binder: RRD/Harrisonburg

©2000 by Prentice-Hall, Inc.
Upper Saddle River, New Jersey 07458

Printed in the United States of America

10 9 8 7 6 5 4 3 2

ISBN 0-8359-5375-0

Prentice-Hall International (UK) Limited, *London*
Prentice-Hall of Australia Pty. Limited, *Sydney*
Prentice-Hall Canada Inc., *Toronto*
Prentice-Hall Hispanoamericana, S.A., *Mexico*
Prentice-Hall of India Private Limited, *New Delhi*
Prentice-Hall Japan, Inc., *Tokyo*
Prentice-Hall (Singapore) Pte. Ltd.
Editora Prentice-Hall do Brasil, Ltda., *Rio de Janeiro*

*To Debbie, Stephen, and Alex for their endless love and
patience throughout this and many other projects.*

E. T. D.

*To my wife, Lori, for her understanding and
support of my many professional endeavors.*

and

*To my parents, Richard and Marie Wieder, and
my sister, Joan, who laid the foundation for my achievements.
My successes belong to the family.*

M. A. W.

CONTENTS

PREFACE

Most firefighters, very early in their training, learn this adage: Take care of yourself first, worry about your partner or the other firefighters second, and make any victims of the incident your third priority. This has been a constant for as long as the fire service has been organized. Even though the widely held public perception is that firefighters will selflessly throw themselves in harm's way to protect a victim, most firefighters realize that that is not necessarily the case. Firefighters cannot help victims if they become victims themselves. When firefighters do become victims, the emergency incident grows in scope and complexity, with firefighters who should be providing care needing help themselves.

Despite being taught this care priority adage, as the rates of fire incidence rose in the 1960s and 1970s, so did the number of firefighter injuries and deaths. Many of these injuries and deaths could be attributed to highly stressed, poorly conditioned firefighters who collapsed after overextending themselves. They and other emergency personnel would get caught up in the action of a major incident and work strenuously for hours on end, never taking a break for rest or nourishment. Too often in such cases, firefighters pushed beyond the point at which their bodies or minds could respond appropriately, resulting in injuries or serious medical emergencies.

As injury and death rates continued to rise, progressive leaders in the fire service realized that changes had to be made. Many fire departments began to take new steps to increase the safety of their firefighters in the early 1980s. Many of the earliest safety improvements could be traced directly back to incidents in which specific problems had occurred. Departments that had bad experiences with hazardous materials incidents formed hazmat teams. Departments that had suffered firefighter injuries or deaths when the firefighters became lost on the fire ground developed accountability programs. Fire departments that had recurring problems with fatigue and stress-related injuries and deaths on the fire ground developed better plans for rotating personnel and getting them the rest, fluids, and nourishment needed to restore them to sound physical condition. Somewhere along the line this last process became known as *Emergency Incident Rehabilitation* or, simply, *rehab*.

Today, the term *rehab* means a specially designated area on the emergency scene where personnel can rest, receive fluids and nourishment, and be evaluated for medical problems. Many jurisdictions routinely operate rehab areas as a part of their overall emergency scene. Correspondingly, the rate of firefighter injuries and deaths due to stress and fatigue has decreased dramatically in recent years.

The inclusion of rehab into emergency operations increased dramatically throughout the nation in the late 1980s in response to the requirements set out in the National Fire Protection Association's (NFPA) Standard 1500, *Standard for Fire*

Department Occupational Safety and Health Program. The first edition of this standard was released in 1987. Although controversial at first, the standard has had a profound positive effect on the safety of firefighters. Departments that had not yet started their own programs used the standard as a template for creating programs that increased the safety of their firefighters. While the standard covered many subjects, both on and off the emergency scene, it was particularly in the area of emergency scene operations that the greatest move forward in safety occurred. Accountability systems, incident management systems, and rehab operations became a normal part of everyday fire department operations.

Many of the ideas discussed in the standard, such as incident management and accountability, received extensive attention and much was written about them. Fire departments looking for guidance on these issues found no shortage of sources.

The issue of rehab operations, on the other hand, received little attention in print. An International Fire Service Training Association (IFSTA) manual or the NFPA *Fire Protection Handbook* devoted a few paragraphs to the topic. The United States Fire Administration released a short sample standard operating procedure (SOP) for rehab operations. Occasionally, an article on rehab appeared in a trade journal, but that was about the extent of coverage. Most fire departments thus had to develop their own SOPs for setting up and carrying out rehab operations at emergency scenes.

The first major step toward adequately addressing the topic of rehab came in 1998 when IFSTA and Brady Publishing formed a joint venture to develop a text for training Emergency Medical Technicians-Basic (EMT-Bs) in the fire service. This book, titled *Fire Service Emergency Care* (FSEC), contains many features that address the special concerns of EMT-Bs operating in a fire department setting. One of these features is an entire chapter on performing rehab operations at the emergency scene. While this information is not a requirement of the U.S. Department of Transportation's national EMT-B curriculum, both IFSTA and Brady felt that the topic was important enough to merit a separate chapter in the book. The response to the chapter and the information contained in it were so positive that FSEC author Dr. Edward Dickinson and IFSTA Senior Editor Mike Wieder decided to expand the information into a book of its own. The document you now hold in your hands is the product of this decision.

This book provides emergency responders with the most comprehensive treatment of Emergency Incident Rehabilitation operations to date. It explores rehab operations in the contexts of both the tactics of fire operations and the provision of medical evaluation and treatment. What the book sets out is not theory, but rather nuts-and-bolts information that can be used by emergency organizations of any size. The information contained in this book will allow departments to meet the intent of NFPA 1500 and is in agreement with the principles of the National Fire Service Incident Management System (IMS). Do note, however, that some of this information may have to be adjusted to satisfy local requirements of particular jurisdictions.

We hope you find this book useful in developing or revising your organization's SOPs for Emergency Incident Rehabilitation. It is everyone's responsibility to ensure the safest possible working conditions for the emergency personnel who operate on the street and in the field. We have tried to do our part by providing this book. We hope that the information in it will help you do your part.

SUGGESTIONS FOR IMPROVEMENTS

Some of the best ideas for training and education methods come from students and instructors who use educational materials in their classes or personnel who are applying in their departments. Any member of the fire or other emergency services who has suggestions for improving this document is encouraged to contact:

Brady Marketing Department
c/o Tiffany Price
Brady/Prentice Hall Health/Pearson Education
One Lake Street
Upper Saddle River, NJ 07458

You may also contact the authors via the Internet. Dr. Dickinson may be reached at:
eddickin@mail.med.upenn.edu

Mike Wieder may be reached at:
mwieder@ifstafpp.okstate.edu

Visit the Brady Website at:
http:/www.bradybooks.com

ACKNOWLEDGMENTS

Our thanks to the reviewers listed below for their feedback and suggestions:

David Daniels
Deputy Chief
Seattle Fire Department
Seattle, Washington

Gary Morris
Assistant Chief
Phoenix Fire Department
Phoenix, Arizona

Michael Mallory
Safety Officer
Tulsa Fire Department
Tulsa, Oklahoma

Gene Chantler
Division Chief, Ret.
Poudre Fire Authority
Fort Collins, Colorado

ABOUT THE AUTHORS

Edward T. Dickinson, M.D., NREMT-P, FACEP, is currently Assistant Professor and Director of EMS Field Operations in the Department of Emergency Medicine, University of Pennsylvania School of Medicine in Philadelphia. He is currently Medical Director of the Malvern Fire Company and of Narberth Ambulance in Pennsylvania. He is also the Medical Director for the town of Colonie, New York, EMS Department and the New York State Police LifeGuard Air Rescue Helicopter program. He is a residency-trained, board-certified emergency medicine physician who is a Fellow of the American College of Emergency Physicians.

He began his career in emergency services in 1979 as a firefighter-EMT in upstate New York. As a volunteer firefighter, he served as a company officer, assistant chief, and training officer. In 1985, he was the first volunteer firefighter in the country to receive the top award for heroism from the *Firehouse Magazine* Heroism and Community Awards program in recognition of his rescue of two elderly women trapped in a house fire.

Dr. Dickinson has remained active in fire and EMS for the past 20 years. He frequently rides with EMS units and has maintained his certification as a National Registry EMT-Paramedic. He has served as medical editor for numerous Brady EMT-B and First Responder texts and is the author of *Fire Service Emergency Care,* an EMT-Basic textbook.

Michael A. Wieder, M.S., CFPS, is currently a senior editor for the International Fire Service Training Association (IFSTA) at Oklahoma State University in Stillwater, Oklahoma. He has written or edited over 20 IFSTA manuals and 100 periodical articles. Mr. Wieder holds an Associate Degree in Fire Technology from Northampton Community College in Bethlehem, Pennsylvania. He also holds a Bachelor's Degree in Fire Protection and Safety Engineering Technology and a Master's Degree in Occupational and Adult Education from Oklahoma State University. A Certified Fire Protection Specialist, he is a principal member of the National Fire Protection Association's Fire Fighter Professional Qualifications (NFPA 1001) committee and serves as secretary of the National Fire Service Incident Management System Consortium. He is a contributing editor to *Firehouse Magazine* and a part-time instructor for Oklahoma State University Fire Service Training. He maintains a very active fire service lecture and legal consultation workload.

Mr. Wieder began his fire service career in 1979 as a volunteer firefighter with the Pennsburg, Pennsylvania, Fire Company. He also served as a volunteer and part-paid firefighter with the Stillwater, Oklahoma, Fire Department.

1

WHAT IS REHAB AND WHY DO WE NEED IT?

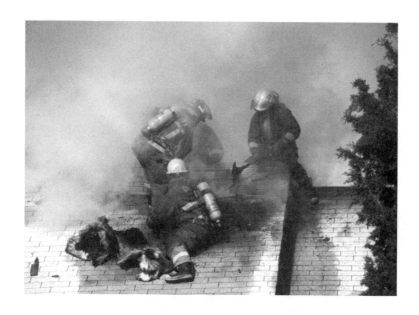

Fire fighting is an inherently hazardous occupation (or avocation for those who volunteer to do it). From the time firefighters leave the fire station or their homes until the time they return, an almost endless variety of hazards await them. Traffic hazards, environmental conditions, products of combustion, the possibilities of trips and falls, bulky protective clothing and equipment, stressful situations, and demanding physical tasks all create difficulties that firefighters must face (Figure 1-1). Anything that will reduce the effects of these dangers, stresses, and physical demands on fire personnel will benefit not only firefighters but their departments as well. In this book, we will explore the role that emergency incident rehabilitation can play in this reduction.

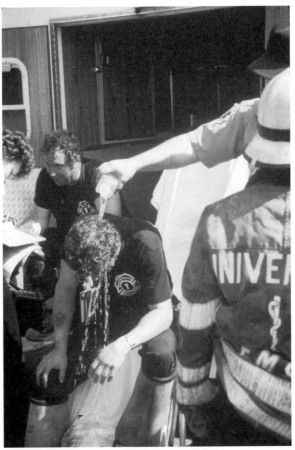

Figure 1-1 Stress, fatigue, or extreme environmental conditions can leave firefighters unable to carry out operational duties.

BACKGROUND TO REHAB

For many years, the fire service treated the element of job-related danger as a badge of courage, worn with pride. Firefighters would boast of this element of danger when discussing the merits of various occupations. The job-related dangers also became a basis for justifying fire department requests for funding or resources to government officials and the public. In many cases, this attitude was rewarded when those requests were granted. Most people have an inherent fear of uncontrolled fire and are apprehensive of getting personally involved in fire fighting and emergency response operations. They are glad that someone else in their community is there to handle these situations.

In the last 20 years or so, however, the attitude of the fire service toward safety has changed dramatically. Firefighters and department officials began to realize that needless deaths and injuries of firefighters were not badges of courage, but indicators of problems. The idea of using injuries and deaths as justification for public support and funding became unacceptable. These changes in attitudes brought with them changes in fire-fighting procedures and policies. As a result, more advances in the area of firefighter safety have probably occurred in the last 20 years than during the entire previous history of organized fire fighting. These advances have led to a nearly 50 percent reduction in firefighter fatalities since the 1970s. Among the most significant of these advances in firefighter safety are the following:

- The development of firefighter professional qualifications standards by the National Professional Qualifications Board (NPQB) and later the National Fire Protection Association (NFPA)
- The development of fire-fighting equipment and apparatus design standards by the NFPA
- The introduction of NFPA 1500, *Standard on Fire Department Occupational Safety and Health Program*, in 1987
- Increased use of incident management systems and firefighter accountability systems at emergency scenes
- Increased awareness of the importance of firefighter fitness and conditioning

The importance of firefighter fitness and conditioning is worth expounding upon. One could argue that, as a whole, today's firefighters are the best physically conditioned ever. Most fire departments and firefighters (particularly those on the career side of the profession) recognize that healthy lifestyles, proper diets, and sound physical conditioning programs are major components of any injury reduction program. No matter how marvelously conditioned firefighters are, however, each has a point after which fatigue and exhaustion reduce effectiveness, increase the likelihood of stress- or fatigue-related illness or injury, and reduce the chance of success of any emergency scene operation. Depending on the environment in which firefighters are working, how well conditioned individual firefighters are, and how strenuous the activity they are performing is, each firefighter will have a different duration of safe operating time.

It would be convenient if every emergency incident ended before any firefighter reached the point at which stress and exhaustion began to compromise his or her safety. And in reality, a high percentage of incidents do end before fatigue becomes a significant problem. However, some incidents extend long beyond the safe operating period for firefighters. Finding safe and effective ways of dealing with these extended incidents continually tests the resourcefulness of fire departments and their personnel.

If firefighters are extended beyond their safe operating periods, the results may be unfortunate:

1. The firefighter may suffer a stress- or fatigue-related illness or injury.
2. The firefighter, although uninjured, will be fatigued to a point at which he or she is unable to continue in the operation and will have to be replaced by another firefighter.
3. The mentally and/or physically fatigued firefighter may make poor decisions in a high-risk environment.

Obviously, any of the previous alternatives is unacceptable. No responsible emergency organization—police, fire, or EMS—can encourage or allow its personnel to exceed their safe operational limits. When a firefighter collapses or is injured, critical resources must be diverted to that firefighter's care. Remember, there is no honor in becoming a liability on the emergency scene. The first goal for any firefighter, career or volunteer, is to return to the fire station or the home in something close to the same condition in which he or she left it.

Wearing personnel down until they are physically unable to continue operations is not much better than leaving them injured or ill. Either alternative produces firefighters who are unable to contribute to the positive resolution of the emergency incident. In addition, if the practice of continually wearing personnel down to this point is followed, the chances of injury or illness to those personnel are greatly increased. Finally, few departments have the luxury of being able to "throw" an unlimited number of firefighters at an incident until it is stabilized. This means that, in addition to a moral obligation to take proper care of personnel operating on the emergency scene, fire departments have practical, tactical reasons for doing so. The help of once-fatigued firefighters may very likely be needed to successfully terminate the incident.

On the other hand, a firefighter who receives adequate rest, nourishment, and medical attention before reaching the "point of no return" will be able to resume emergency scene operations and make effective decisions. How to achieve this outcome is the subject of the remainder of this book. During extended operations, it is necessary to recognize when firefighters need to take a break and to optimize the chances that the break will restore the firefighters to full effectiveness. The firefighters must be allowed enough time to overcome their fatigue, to be checked by medical personnel, and to receive replenishment of fluids and nourishment necessary to continue in the operation.

In this respect, fire fighting is not that unlike organized team sports. In fact, over the years many fire instructors have made comparisons between fire fighting and football. Both activities involve groups of properly conditioned and equipped players. Strategy and tactics are necessary to carry out the game plan. If an offensive strategy is not successful, the team—firefighters or football players—must revert to a defensive stop strategy. Each individual has a role within the orchestrated play of the entire team on the scene or on the field.

Parallels between the activities break down when players and firefighters become tired. When football players are tired, the coach can call a time-out or pull players to the sidelines for a breather. Unfortunately, incident commanders generally do not have the luxury of calling a time-out on the emergency scene. The incident would progress during any operational downtime, making downtime unacceptable. Simply put, you cannot call a time-out on an emergency scene. Thus, it becomes important to find a way to get some players (firefighters) over to the sidelines when they need a rest while still maintaining an operationally effective number of personnel to deal with the incident. This process is known as *emergency incident rehabilitation* (EIR), or simply *rehab*. The rehab area is the emergency scene's "sideline."

While the focus of this manual is clearly on firefighters, it must be noted that the principles of sound rehab procedures apply to all other types of emergency responders as well. These may include law-enforcement officials, emergency medical personnel, public utility workers, private hazardous materials mitigation personnel, and any other individuals who commonly assist at emergency scenes. Because the fire department is typically more practiced in proper rehab procedures, its personnel often assume a lead role in the rehabbing of all emergency responders at an incident.

WHAT IS REHAB?

The term *rehabilitation*, or *rehab*, has had many different applications. It has been used to describe processes such as these:

- Fixing up old houses
- Providing posthospital care for injured or ill people
- Providing substance abuse treatment

Although it is possible to develop parallels between these applications and fire service use of the term, the fit is not exact. More closely related to the fire service's idea of rehabilitation is the dictionary definition that says, "to restore or bring to a condition of health or useful and constructive activity." In the fire service, *rehabilitation,* or *rehab,* describes the process of providing rest, rehydration, nourishment, and medical evaluation to responders who are involved in extended and/or extreme incident scene operations. The goal of the process is getting the responders either back into the action or back to the station safely. Proper rehab operations assure that the physical and mental conditions of responders operating at the emergency scene do not deteriorate to a point that affects the safety of any responder or that jeopardizes the safety and integrity of the operation.

Note that rehab operations are not limited to *emergency* scenes. Any type of activity that involves the extended presence of firefighters and other emergency workers may necessitate rehab operations. Other types of activities that might necessitate rehab operations include the following:

- Training exercises
- Athletic events
- Parade or event standbys

Textbook definitions are nice, but rehab can also be described in simpler, more practical terms. In practical terms, we can say that rehab is a part of an overall emergency scene effort in which firefighters who are exhausted, thirsty, hungry, medically compromised, and perhaps emotionally upset are restored to something close to the same condition they were in before responding to the call. Although fire fighting is a physically demanding business, it is not—or should not be—a masochistic or sadistic one. Fire departments have professional and moral obligations to take care of their own people in a responsible manner.

WHY DO WE NEED REHAB?

In order to develop an effective strategy for providing emergency incident rehabilitation, it is important to understand the reasons that rehab is necessary. As stated earlier, fire fighting and rescue work are dangerous. A review of injury and death statistics associated with the fire service will help to point up just how dangerous. These statistics, along with other factors cited below, will clarify the need to establish effective emergency incident rehabilitation procedures.

Injury and Death Statistics

In the United States, the NFPA maintains the most comprehensive firefighter injury and death statistics. At the time of this book's publication, the latest statistics available were from calendar year 1996. In that year, the NFPA reported that slightly more than 87,000 firefighters were injured during the performance of their duties. During the same period, 92 firefighters died as a direct result of fire department activities.

Table 1-1 provides a breakdown of the types of injuries suffered by firefighters and the types of duties they were performing at the time of injury. The table does not specifically show injuries that occurred as a result of overfatigue. It should be noted, however, that injuries caused by heart attacks, strokes, strains, sprains, and thermal stress accounted for about 50 percent of all firefighter injuries. It can rationally be assumed that a significant portion of these injuries occurred when firefighters were overfatigued.

Table 1-1 Firefighter Injuries by Nature of Injury and Type of Duty (1996)

Nature of Injury	Responding to or Returning from an Incident		Fireground		Nonfire Emergency		Training		Other On-duty		Totals	
	Number	Percent	Number	Percent	Number	Percent	Number	Percent	Number	Percent	Number	Percent
Burns (fire or chemical)	65	1.0	4,360	9.5	140	1.1	635	10.2	215	1.3	5,415	6.2
Smoke or gas inhalation	115	1.8	4,660	10.2	305	2.4	70	1.1	105	0.6	5,255	6.0
Other respiratory distress	45	0.7	740	1.6	210	1.6	75	1.2	125	0.8	1,195	1.4
Eye irritation	225	3.6	2,735	6.0	390	3.1	165	2.7	620	3.8	4,135	4.7
Wound (cut, bleeding, bruise)	1,375	21.8	8,775	19.2	2,055	16.3	1,085	17.5	3,325	20.4	16,615	19.1
Dislocation, fracture	190	3.0	1,090	2.4	260	2.0	235	3.8	550	3.4	2,325	2.7
Heart attack or stroke	25	0.4	300	0.7	45	0.4	35	0.6	310	1.9	715	0.8
Strain, sprain, muscular pain	3,545	56.1	17,455	38.2	7,020	55.6	3,160	51.0	8,540	52.5	39,720	45.6
Thermal stress (frostbite, heat exhaustion)	60	1.0	2,270	5.9	185	1.5	260	4.2	100	0.6	3,325	3.8
Other	670	10.6	2,890	6.3	2,020	16.0	480	7.7	2,390	14.7	8,450	9.7
Totals	6,315		45,725		12,630		6,200		16,280		87,150	

When reviewing the death statistics, the effects of stress on the firefighter become even more clear. The records for 1996 indicate that some 47 of the 93 deaths were attributed to heart attacks and strokes (Table 1-2). This means that *about 50 percent of all firefighter deaths were, to some extent, directly attributed to stress and overexertion.*

The NFPA has received medical documentation on 532 of the 1,078 firefighter heart attack fatalities over the past 20 years. Those records included some interesting facts:

- 49.6 percent of the victims had had previous heart attacks or bypass surgery.
- 32.7 percent had severe arteriosclerotic heart disease.
- 11.7 percent had hypertension or diabetes.

When looking at both the injury and death statistics together, another interesting fact emerges. While heart attacks accounted for only 0.8 percent (715 incidents) of all firefighter *injuries* in 1996, they were responsible for about 50 percent (46 incidents) of all *deaths*. Thus, about 6 percent of all heart attack injuries are likely to be fatal, while 0.05 percent of all other fireground illnesses or injuries are fatal. This means that a firefighter who suffers a heart attack on the fireground is *125 times more likely to die* than a firefighter who suffers some other type of injury.

The Impact of Deaths and Injuries

There is little question that firefighter deaths and injuries deeply impact the firefighters, their loved ones, and their fire departments. On a personal level, a stress-related injury may limit a firefighter's ability to make a living in the future. This is true both for career firefighters and for volunteers, who may be unable to return to

Table 1-2   Nature of Fatal Injuries (1996)

Nature of Injury	*Number of Deaths*
Heart attack	46
Internal trauma	20
Asphyxiation	6
Gunshot	5
Crushing	5
Burns	3
Electrocution	3
Stroke (CVA)	1
Drowning	1
Heat stroke	1
Hemorrhaging	1
Other	1

their primary place of employment. Injury may also limit promotional opportunities if it prevents a firefighter from working "in the line" operations. These disabling injuries can also affect an individual's ability to perform other activities he or she may have enjoyed prior to the disability. One incidence of overexertion can thus have lifelong consequences, even if it is not fatal.

The hardships that result for family members and friends of firefighters who suffer stress-related injuries and deaths go without saying.

Firefighter deaths and injuries also have measurable impacts on fire departments, both from an immediate tactical standpoint and from a long-term standpoint. The downing of a firefighter on the emergency scene adds significant additional tactical considerations to an already complicated situation. Personnel must to be assigned to treat and transport the downed firefighter (Figure 1-2). Additional personnel must

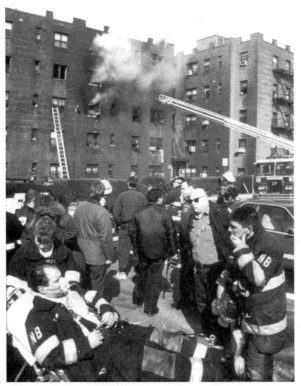

Figure 1-2 Whenever firefighters are placed out of service by injury or illness at the emergency scene, other personnel must be assigned to treat and transport them.

take over the functions that were being carried out by the downed firefighter, his crew, and the rescuers who are providing aid for the stricken member. All things considered, a single downed firefighter can increase the staffing levels needed to handle a routine single-family-dwelling fire by as much as 50 percent.

Beyond its impact on the immediate incident, the loss of a firefighter to death or debilitating injury has a long-term effect on the fire department. A career department will have to hire and train a new firefighter to replace the lost one. A volunteer fire department, which may already be short on personnel, will lose a valuable resource to the department that may not be easily replaced. In addition, the deaths or debilitating injuries of members of the department will affect the morale of both career and volunteer firefighters.

Simply stated, then, the failure to take good care of firefighters on any emergency incident can result in severe hardships for many people. As you will read, many of the situations that cause these hardships could be easily avoided with a little bit of planning combined with a little bit of common sense.

The Impact of NFPA 1500

It is safe to say that few things have more positively affected the well-being of members of the North American fire service in the last 50 years than the introduction of NFPA 1500, *Standard on Fire Department Occupational Safety and Health Program,* in 1987. At the time it was adopted, many fire service people feared that NFPA 1500 would have negative consequences for fire departments. Some people even forecast that smaller departments would be forced to close their doors because they would be unable to meet its requirements. In general, time has proved these fears to be unfounded. Most of the consequences resulting from the imposition of the standard on fire departments have proved to be positive. To date, there have been no documented cases of a fire department "going out of business" because of the standard.

Before going any further, it is important to briefly address the difference between laws and standards. *Laws* are rules of conduct for a society that are legally adopted by a government. There are criminal consequences for failure to obey a law. If you get caught exceeding a posted speed limit, you get a ticket and pay a fine. If you get caught robbing a bank, you go to jail.

Standards are consensus positions on some aspects of a particular area or discipline that are developed by a group of people with a common interest in that area or discipline. Unless formally adopted into law by a governmental body, there is no criminal penalty for failing to obey a standard. However, in the case of NFPA standards, civil courts have recognized them as nationally accepted practices. Thus, while failure to establish a rehab area at an emergency scene may not lead to a prison term, failure to establish such an area may lead to civil liability for the department. In other words, the department might be sued and forced to pay monetary damages for "failure to meet accepted standards of practice." This is the impetus for most fire departments to follow NFPA standards.

Section 6-6, "Rehabilitation During Emergency Operations," of NFPA 1500 (1997 edition) is dedicated solely to the topic of emergency incident rehabilitation. The objectives contained in this section include the following:

6-6.1* The fire department shall develop standard operating guidelines that outline a systematic approach for the rehabilitation of members operating at incidents. Provisions addressed in this guideline shall include medical evaluation and treatment, food and fluid replenishment, crew rotation, and relief from extreme climatic conditions.

A-6-6.1 Having a pre-planned rehabilitation program that is applicable to most incident types is essential for the health and safety of members. The rehabilitation plan should outline an on-going rehabilitation for simple or short-duration incidents as well as a process to transition into the rehabilitation needs of a large or long-term incident. Medical evaluation and treatment in the on-scene rehabilitation area should be conducted according to EMS protocols developed by the fire department in consultation with the fire department physician and the EMS medical director. If ALS personnel are available, this level of EMS care is preferred.

6-6.2* The incident commander shall consider the circumstances of each incident and initiate rest and rehabilitation in accordance with the standard operating guidelines, and NFPA 1561 *Standard on Fire Department Incident Management System.*

A-6-6.2 Weather factors during emergency incidents can impact severely on the safety and health of members, particularly during extremes of heat and cold. Where these factors combine with long-duration incidents or situations that require heavy exertion, the risks to members increase rapidly. The fire department should develop procedures, in consultation with the fire department physician, to provide relief from adverse climatic conditions.

Typical rehabilitation considerations for operations during hot weather extremes are: (1) moving fatigued or unassigned personnel away from the hazardous area of the incident; (2) removal of personal protective equipment; (3) ensuring that personnel are out of direct sunlight; (4) ensuring that there is adequate air movement over personnel, either naturally or mechanically; (5) providing personnel with fluid replenishment, especially water; and (6) providing medical evaluation for personnel showing signs or symptoms of heat exhaustion or heat stroke.

Typical rehabilitation considerations for operations during cold weather extremes are: (1) moving fatigued or unassigned personnel away from the hazardous area of the incident; (2) providing shelter from wind and temperature extremes; (3) providing personnel with fluid replenishment, especially water; and (4) providing medical evaluation for personnel showing signs or symptoms of frostbite, hypothermia, or other cold-related injury.

6-6.3* Such on-scene rehabilitation shall include at least basic life-support care.

A-6-6.3 The assignment of an ambulance or other support crew to the rehabilitation function is essential during long-duration or heavy exertion incident operations. This crew can assist with rehabilitation functions as well as be available to provide immediate life-support needs for members.

6-6.4 Each member operating at an incident shall be responsible to communicate rehabilitation and rest needs to their supervisor.

In addition to providing objectives for rehab, NFPA 1500 covers a wide variety of other safety considerations pertaining to emergency operations as well as to routine fire department activities. Sections on topics such as physical conditioning programs, stress counseling, training, and apparatus safety provide sound advice to fire departments that are seeking to improve safety for their personnel.

Most departments have tried to address as many requirements of NFPA 1500 as they reasonably can. The effects of their efforts are now becoming visible. In the 10 years preceding the adoption of the first edition of NFPA 1500, an average of 60 firefighters a year died of heart attacks. In the period from 1991 through 1996, this figure dropped to an average of 42 a year. While 42 deaths a year is still too many, that average represents a decrease of almost 33 percent in deaths caused by heart attacks. On a similar note, the total number of fireground injuries in 1987 numbered 57,755. By 1996, that number had dropped to 45,725 (a 21 percent decline). The improvements to fire department health and safety programs and the corresponding reduction in casualties result, at least in part, from the influence of NFPA 1500.

THE FUNCTIONS OF A REHAB OPERATION

In order to develop a standard procedure for providing on-scene firefighter rehabilitation, it is important to understand the seven basic functions of any emergency incident rehabilitation operation. All seven of these functions must be accounted for when developing standard operating procedures (SOPs) for rehab. The seven basic EIR functions include the following (Figure 1-3):

1. Physical assessment
2. Revitalization (rest, rehydration, and nutritional support)
3. Medical evaluation and treatment
4. Continual monitoring of physical condition
5. Transportation for those requiring treatment at a hospital
6. Initial critical incident stress assessment and support
7. Reassignment

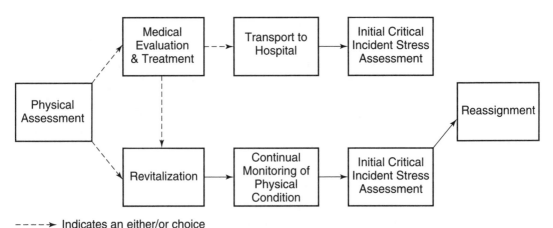

- - - - → Indicates an either/or choice

Figure 1-3 The basic functions provided by emergency incident rehabilitation.

Physical Assessment

The first function that must be carried out when any firefighter enters the rehab area is a general physical assessment of his or her well-being. A determination needs to be made about whether the firefighter is tired, hurt, upset, thirsty, or hungry. Once the person's status has been determined, he or she can be initially directed to the most-needed rehab services. Basic vital signs of all persons entering rehab should be taken at this point. Obviously, if firefighters are ill or injured, medical evaluation and treatment are the top priorities. If firefighters are simply tired, thirsty, and hungry, these needs can be immediately addressed. If, after the minimum stay in rehab mandated by department SOPs, firefighters meet the criteria for returning to service, they can be sent on their way (following formal reassignment procedures).

Revitalization

The most commonly performed function in the rehab area, other than the physical assessment that everyone should undergo, is revitalization of firefighters who have entered the area. Revitalization is not a high-tech procedure. The three basic needs that are met during revitalization are rest, fluid replenishment, and nutrition. Firefighters should be allowed to rest long enough for their body core temperatures and vital signs to return to an acceptable level. If they are too hot, they must be cooled down. If they are too cold, they must be warmed up. They should be provided with appropriate fluids to replace those lost during their period of heavy work (Figure 1-4). If they are hungry, they should receive nutritionally sound food. (Fluid and nutrition replacement will be discussed in detail in Chapter 5.)

Medical Evaluation and Treatment

Firefighters who appear to be ill or injured should be assigned to personnel in the medical evaluation/treatment area of rehab. This assignment should not be delayed by providing the firefighters with drinks or food, unless medical evaluation shows this to be a priority. (Information on who should perform the medical evaluations is covered in Chapter 3. Information on how to evaluate and treat firefighters requiring attention is covered in detail in Chapter 4.)

Continual Monitoring of Physical Condition

Once firefighters are in the rehab area for either rest or medical attention, their conditions must be monitored. Most firefighters assigned to rehab will show signs of improvement fairly rapidly. If they improve enough to meet the criteria for release from rehab (discussed in Chapter 4), they are ready for reassignment or to return to quarters. Firefighters who do not respond to rest or medical attention will require more intensive interventions. No one should be released from rehab until he or she

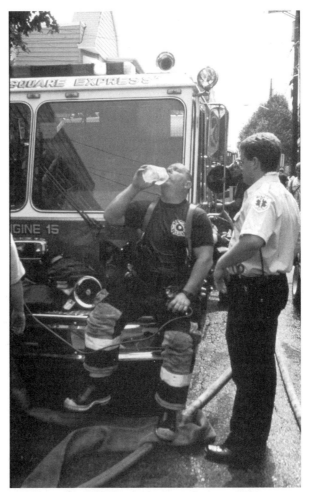

Figure 1-4   Rehydration, the replacement of body fluids, is one of the most important functions in rehab.

is medically and physically sound or is to be transported to a medical facility for further treatment.

Transportation for Those Requiring Treatment at a Hospital

Firefighters who do not respond to actions taken in the rehab area, who are injured, or who meet other medically based criteria should be transported to a medical facility for further evaluation and treatment. Part of the overall rehab SOPs must detail who will do the transporting. In most cases, it is advisable to send the firefighter in an ambulance, either the fire department's own or one from a separate EMS agency. Doing this allows appropriate care to be taken in case the person's condition worsens en route to the hospital. SOPs should also call for an appropriate number of ambulances to be standing by at the rehab area or in a nearby staging area. The actual number will vary depending upon the nature of the incident and the number of personnel operating on the scene.

Initial Critical Incident Stress Assessment and Support

In recent years, the emotional aspects of providing emergency service have gained increasing attention. Emergency service providers confront, on a regular basis, some of the most demanding and difficult situations people can face. On some emergency calls, no amount of training or equipment will be able to help a victim. This is very frustrating for responders. Over time, the cumulative effects of such calls will take a toll on almost everyone, eventually producing unacceptable levels of stress. In some cases, a high level of stress results, not from cumulative effects, but rather from a single critical incident that affects the responder in a greater than normal manner, producing an extreme stress reaction.

In the 1970s, the fire service began to recognize the importance of dealing with these incidents through *critical incident stress debriefing* (CISD). Many organizations have implemented procedures and provided personnel to deal with critical incident stress both on the emergency scene and in follow-up care long after the incident has been formally terminated. On major incidents where critical incident stress is likely, or even on smaller incidents where personnel are showing signs of problems, CISD operations should be initiated. The logical place to locate these operations on the fireground and in the Incident Management System is within the rehab area. (More information on CISD procedures is provided in Chapter 4.)

Reassignment

Once firefighters have been restored to acceptable physical and emotional condition, they are ready to be either reassigned to the incident or sent back to their quarters. Each department will have its own procedures for how this process works. Chapter 3 contains general information on how reassignment can be accomplished in a tactically sound manner.

SUGGESTED READINGS

Foley, Steven, ed. *NFPA 1500 Handbook*. Quincy, MA: National Fire Protection Association, 1998.

National Fire Protection Association. *NFPA 1500, Standard for Fire Department Occupational Safety and Health Program*. Quincy, MA: National Fire Protection Association, 1997.

Wieder, Michael A., ed. *Fire Department Occupational Safety*. Stillwater, OK: International Fire Service Training Association, 1992.

2

KNOWING WHEN TO ESTABLISH REHAB AND UNDERSTANDING ITS ROLE IN THE INCIDENT MANAGEMENT SYSTEM

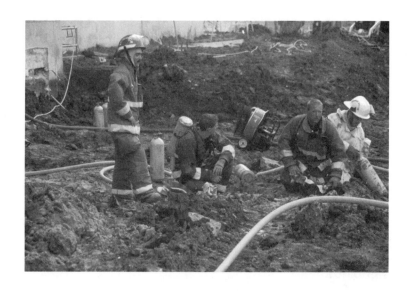

A key consideration in emergency incident rehabilitation is exactly *when* to establish rehab operations at an emergency incident. Waiting too long to recognize the effects of fatigue on personnel and to develop a plan for dealing with those effects puts the Incident Commander in an operational hole that may be impossible to climb out of as the incident progresses. The Incident Commander must be able to recognize the need for rehab in a timely manner and see that a plan of action is put into motion.

Once the decision to implement the rehab function has been made, the next issue that must be considered is how that sector/group will fit into the incident management system (IMS) that is in place. All responders must be familiar with the IMS used in their jurisdiction. Personnel who do not understand the IMS are most likely to operate outside it, which, as you will read, can create many hazards for emergency personnel. Most IMS plans used in the fire and EMS communities today have defined places for rehab operations. Personnel assigned to Rehab must understand how their "piece of the puzzle" fits into the overall IMS structure.

An additional issue that involves both IMS in general and rehab operations in particular is that of the accountability of personnel operating on the emergency scene. Far too frequently, fireground operations have failed to account for the location of all emergency workers. Such failures have led to situations in which firefighters went unaccounted for following structural collapses or the appearance of other unanticipated hazards. In the hectic minutes and hours that followed, no one recognized that personnel were missing. Failures to track the whereabouts of personnel in these incidents led to delayed, unfocused rescue operations and the loss of the lives of emergency personnel. Such incidents have prompted many fire departments to improve their tracking of emergency scene personnel, making sure the assignment or position of every emergency worker is documented at all times. Because rehab is one of the areas to which firefighters are assigned during emergency operations, responders staffing Rehab must understand how their department's accountability system operates and must make sure that all personnel in Rehab strictly adhere to accountability procedures. In other words, the accountability system must be able to note that emergency personnel have left the operational area and have entered Rehab.

WHEN TO ESTABLISH REHAB

The goal of emergency incident rehabilitation operations is to lessen the risks of injury that may result from extended incident operations, which are sometimes carried out under adverse conditions involving weather and other factors. Ideally, rehab operations should commence whenever emergency operations pose the risk of pushing personnel beyond a safe level of physical or mental endurance. However, determining exactly what that level is, and what types or combinations of incidents, conditions, and time frames require the establishment of Rehab, is not so clear.

There is no law or standard that sets out specific criteria for the establishment of rehab operations. Commonly, a variety of factors, when considered as a whole, will make the need for a Rehab group/sector apparent. In most cases, the establishment of Rehab is a judgment call made by the Incident Commander. Ideally, the establishment of Rehab should be a routine, proactive measure rather than a reactive response made as firefighters begin to collapse.

Some guidelines that Incident Commanders should consider when deciding whether to establish rehab operations on emergency scenes are discussed below. Note that these guidelines are not definitive statements about when and when not to establish Rehab. Each emergency incident involves different conditions and therefore will have different requirements. The Incident Commander and other personnel must use their experiences and make careful observations about scene conditions when deciding whether or not to establish Rehab. For example, company officers should provide feedback to the Command post when they detect of levels of fatigue among their crew(s) sufficient to warrant establishment of Rehab.

Extended Fire Incidents

Perhaps the most common situations that should trigger the establishment of Rehab operations are extended fire-fighting operations. While the types of fire incidents that could last long enough for the establishment of a Rehab group/sector are varied and many, only the three most common will be discussed here. These situations include:

- Structure fires
- High-rise structural fires
- Wildland fires

Structure Fires

The classic National Fire Protection Association definition of *structural fire fighting* is "the activities of rescue, fire suppression, and property conservation involving buildings, enclosed structures, vehicles, vessels, aircraft, or like properties that are involved in a fire or emergency situation." This broad definition extends beyond what most firefighters have traditionally associated with fire fighting. Clearly, fires involving things such as ships, aircraft, and large or multiple vehicles can be long-term incidents that will require the rehabilitation of personnel operating on the scene. In most jurisdictions, however, the likelihood of one of those incidents (other than a multiple-vehicle fire, such as might occur in a wrecking yard) is rather slim. This discussion, therefore, will focus on the more common types of structure fires that most fire departments routinely face.

A common rule of thumb for requiring a firefighter to enter Rehab for evaluation is exhaustion of two standard 30-minute, self-contained breathing apparatus (SCBA) cylinders or one 60-minute cylinder. In either of these instances, a firefighter will probably have been engaged in strenuous work for about 45 minutes.

Incident Commanders should keep this rule in mind when trying to determine the need to begin rehab activities.

Firefighters should always wear SCBA in any environment where they are, or have the potential to be, exposed to heat, smoke, and toxic gases from a fire. These situations include both interior and exterior fire-fighting operations. SCBA should also be worn during *all* facets of interior fire-fighting operations, including rescue, fire suppression, and property conservation. Historically, firefighters have been quick to remove their SCBA when performing property conservation (more commonly referred to as *salvage and overhaul*) functions (Figure 2-1). Research has indicated, however, that extremely high levels of carbon monoxide and other dangerous gases are often present in structures during this period. Firefighters should continue breathing through SCBA until the atmosphere has been tested and proved safe

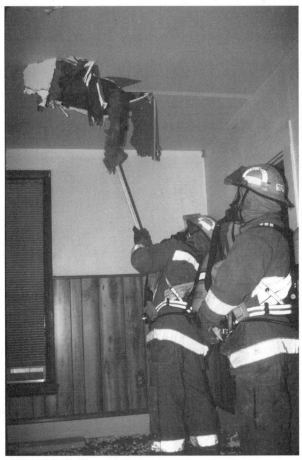

Figure 2-1   Salvage and overhaul operations can involve physical stresses that will require the establishment of rehab operations.

or until absolutely no more smoke or steam is present. Each jurisdiction should establish a standard operating procedure that defines the level of carbon monoxide below which SCBA may be removed.

In addition, crew members should remain alert for symptoms of carbon monoxide poisoning, which include headache, nausea, dizziness, confusion or inability to think clearly, convulsions, and unresponsiveness. What may appear to be extreme exhaustion may, in fact, be CO poisoning. Firefighters should be able to recognize this situation and retreat from it for rehabilitation.

The Incident Commander must keep the information in the previous paragraphs in mind when estimating the duration of an incident and determining the need for rehab operations. In some cases, the rescue and fire suppression activities may be completed in a matter of minutes. However, the property conservation activities could take an hour or more. A quick "knockdown" time does not necessarily mean that there is no need to establish rehab. The hardest part of the incident might be just beginning at that point.

The Incident Commander should also keep in mind that overall rehab needs for the incident may change as the incident evolves. For example, suppose the decision is made to launch an aggressive, offensive, interior attack on a well-advanced fire within a large structure. A large number of personnel will be required for this attack. These personnel will be operating under extremely exhausting conditions and will require extensive rehab when they have reached their limits. A large-scale Rehab group/sector—possibly more than one—will be needed to handle all the personnel. As this incident progresses, suppose that, for safety reasons, the Incident Commander decides to abandon the interior attack and convert to a defensive exterior operation. At this point, all personnel will be removed from the building. Large-volume master stream devices will be set up outside the building and a "surround-and-drown" operation will commence (Figure 2-2). Once the master stream devices are set up and flowing, there would generally be little for the firefighters to do but stand by and watch. Obviously, this will be less stressful than the initial fire attack. At this point, it may be possible for the Incident Commander to scale down rehab operations.

Finally, even at minor structure fires, accommodations should be made for some form of rehab, even at the company level. In these cases, the establishment of a formal rehab area may not be necessary, but a cooler of water or a sports drink should be accessible. The availability of rehydration in such cases enhances firefighters' comfort and helps keep their body fluids at acceptable levels.

High-Rise Structural Fires

A high-rise structure can usually be defined as a multistoried structure of a height greater than 75 feet (23 meters). However, some buildings less than 75 feet (23 meters) tall present the same problems as those that height or taller. Frequently those buildings constructed just short of code requirements for high-rise structures do not have all the same fire protection and safety features of buildings that meet

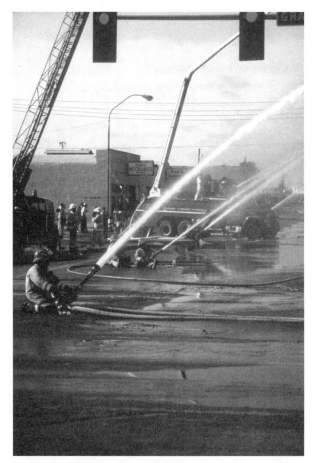

Figure 2-2   During a "surround-and-drown" operation, it may be possible to scale back rehab operations.

the high-rise code. This increases risks and difficulties for firefighters operating in those buildings.

Two basic aspects of high-rise fire-fighting pose exceptional challenges from the standpoint of firefighter rehabilitation. One challenge is the highly strenuous nature of the work involved in fighting these fires. To start with, firefighters often must expend large amounts of energy simply to reach the location of the fire. It may not be possible to take elevators to the fire floor or even near it (Figure 2-3). This means that firefighters, wearing heavy personal protective equipment, must carry all their fire-fighting equipment to the fire. Depending on how high in the structure firefighters must climb, they could be in need of rehab even before actual fire-fighting activities begin.

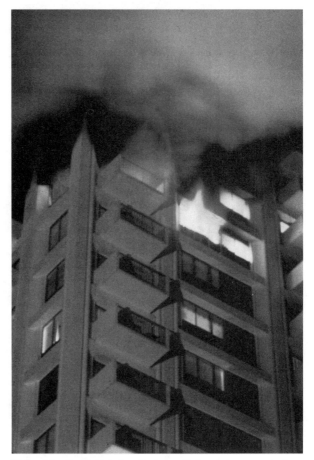

Figure 2-3 Fires in high-rise structures will almost always require the establishment of rehab operations.

Once the location of the fire is reached, firefighters will often face extreme high-temperature conditions because the ability to vent the fire area is limited. Deployment of hose streams and performance of other normally routine fire-fighting tactics will be more difficult than the same tasks carried out in a ground-level structure. As a rule, the extra expenditure of energy by firefighters in these situations means that rehab operations will be required early in the incident.

The second aspect of high-rise fire-fighting that poses a challenge for rehab operations is the large number of firefighters that are commonly needed in such incidents. Because the work is so strenuous, multiple companies of personnel are often needed to perform tasks that a single company could handle at a routine house fire.

It is a commonly used rule of thumb for Incident Commanders to plan to use *three* companies to perform each facet of a high-rise fire operation. For example, suppose it is necessary to deploy a 1¾-inch (45-millimeter) handline for fire attack. In a routine house fire, a single company could easily handle the deployment and use of the hose line. When the same handline is deployed on an upper floor in a high-rise structure, however, the Incident Commander should assign three companies to the job. To ensure that the handline is in continuous operation, at any given time, the three companies assigned to it will be deployed as follows:

- One company will be operating the handline in the fire area.
- One company will be standing by ready outside the stairwell door leading to the location where the handline is being operated.
- One company will be in the staging area two floors below the fire floor. The firefighters in this company will be replacing their air cylinders and making other preparations necessary to be ready to return to the fire floor.

The large number of very fatigued firefighters likely to be found at high-rise fires demands that a sound rehab plan be implemented early in the incident. *Tiered rehab operations* may be necessary at these incidents. Tiered operations are those in which some basic rehab functions are performed at a forward location in the fire building near the fire floor, while other, more extensive rehab is being performed at a location farther from the fire.

Before giving an example of a tiered rehab operation, it is necessary to explain how the term *staging* is used for high-rise fire-fighting operations. Traditional fire service use of this term refers to the practice of parking responding fire companies some distance away from the emergency scene where they await orders for deployment from the Incident Commander. In high-rise fire-fighting operations, staging refers to a safe area, preferably two floors below the fire floor where extra equipment and personnel are assembled to support the attack. All personnel who ascend the building to assist with operations must check in at staging and wait for assignment. Personnel who are relieved from forward operating positions report back to staging for equipment replenishment, rest, and reassignment.

Personnel who are in staging are still in service and not subject to extensive rehab procedures there. However, minor rehab functions may be performed at this location. Water or other fluid replenishment drinks should be provided at staging. Personnel should also be observed for excessive stress and fatigue and sent to the formal rehab area if necessary. Beyond those functions, most of the traditional functions of rehab will not be performed at staging.

A formal rehab area—perhaps more than one—should be established at a location near the forward staging area. Depending on the size of the structure, incident conditions, and local department SOPs, the rehab area may be on the same floor as the staging area, on a floor below it, or completely outside the fire building. Keep in mind that if rehab and the formal staging area are on the same floors, they must be maintained as two separate and distinct functions. Personnel in staging and personnel in rehab are not interchangeable. Personnel who are fit enough to leave rehab may then be assigned to the staging area. However, personnel should never proceed directly from rehab to a forward operating position. This defeats the accountability and organizational benefits provided by the staging area.

Wildland Fires

Wildland fires involve natural cover fuels, including grasses, weeds, agricultural crops, shrubs, and trees. Wildland fire incidents range from small fires that involve only several square yards or meters of fuel to enormously large fires that cover more than 100,000 acres and last for days or weeks. Although aircraft and other equipment are used in combating wildland fires, the primary method of attack still involves heavy manual labor by large numbers of specially trained firefighters (Figure 2-4).

Firefighters in wildland fires typically work 12- to 24-hour shifts on the fireline, usually in high atmospheric temperatures, sometimes in high humidity, and sometimes at high elevations. Just as there is less oxygen available to support a fire at higher elevations, there is less oxygen for hard-working firefighters to breathe. In addition, firefighters may have to reach the elevation of the fireline on foot and to construct a scratch line (unfinished preliminary control line) along the way. They may arrive at the fireline already physically exhausted and dehydrated.

All these factors—in addition to the normal fatigue that results from doing hard work in adverse circumstances—combine to create conditions in which firefighters become very vulnerable to stress- and heat-related problems. These conditions take a terrific toll on even the fittest firefighters, and those who are in less-than-ideal condition suffer even more.

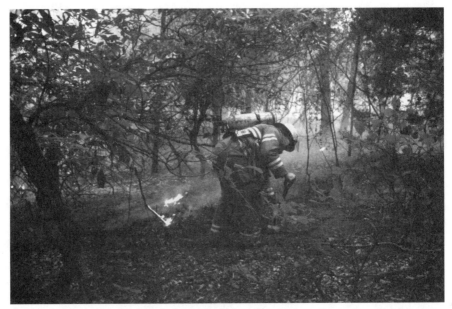

Figure 2-4   Firefighters responding to wildland fires can experience severe physical stress from the nature of the work and the environmental conditions.

On large-scale incidents, the Incident Commander should consider setting up one or more Rehab stations or camps to reduce the loss of fire-fighting personnel to stress, fatigue, and injuries. These stations provide firefighters with shade, water and other fluids, and first aid if needed. Remember, however, that under typical fire-line conditions, firefighters should be encouraged to pace themselves, take frequent short breaks, drink plenty of water, and monitor each other for signs of physical distress.

Incident Commanders will have to use good judgment when determining whether rehab operations are needed at wildland fires. A number of factors must be considered, including the following:

- *The size of the fire and the length of time that will be required until termination of the incident.* Obviously, large fires require more time to control and will be likely candidates for establishment of rehab operations. Generally speaking, fires that will involve heavy manual labor for more than 1 hour are likely to require some type of rehab operation.
- *The weather conditions at the time of the fire.* The hotter and more humid the weather is, the more fatiguing the labor will be to firefighters.
- *The elevation above sea level at which the fire is located.* As mentioned earlier, fires that occur at high altitudes will require greater expenditures of energy by firefighters because of reduced levels of atmospheric oxygen and other factors than will fires closer to sea level.
- *The method of attack employed by firefighters.* The amount of fatigue experienced by firefighters will vary with the type of work they are doing. Firefighters who are riding an apparatus during pump-and-roll operations are not apt to tire as quickly as those who are constructing a firebreak with hand tools.

Agencies that routinely handle large wildland fires typically have established SOPs that dictate when rehab operations should be established. These guidelines also indictate where rehab areas should be set up and how often personnel should be rotated through them. Incident Commanders must evaluate the operational factors described above in conjunction with agency SOPs so that rehab operations are established early enough in the incident to benefit the initial responders on the scene.

Hazardous Material Incidents

A *hazardous material* (hazmat) is any substance, in any form or quantity, that poses an unreasonable risk to safety, health, and property when transported, used, or stored. A hazardous material incident can then be defined as the release, or potential release, of a hazardous material from its container into the environment. Hazardous material incidents pose extraordinary challenges for emergency responders because often the exact nature of the material is unknown in the early stages of the incident. Responders must, therefore, take maximum precautions while they determine the material involved and implement a strategy to mitigate the incident's effects.

Hazmat workers must perform a slow, thorough investigation of the problem, often wearing heavy, totally encapsulating protective garments. The process of donning the protective garments, moving to the hazmat location, performing the necessary work, returning to a safe area for decontamination, and doffing the equipment is an arduous one (Figure 2-5). While in the protective clothing, the wearer relies on air from an SCBA for survival. The construction of the protective garments keeps hazardous materials from getting to the worker; at the same time, those garments prevent heat and perspiration generated by the wearer from dissipating. Thus, even short-term hazmat incidents can result in excessive stress to emergency responders. These effects are further compounded in hot and humid weather conditions.

Once an Incident Commander determines that a reported hazmat incident will involve placing personnel in totally encapsulating protective clothing, provisions for responder rehab should be set in motion immediately. The rehab area must be in place and ready to accept responders as soon as the first crews are decontaminated and have removed their protective clothing. The rehab area must be located upwind of the incident and in the cold zone. Considerations for the siting of rehab areas are covered in more detail in Chapter 3.

Some hazmat incidents may not require the special protective clothing described above. An example of such an incident would be an overturned, leaking gasoline tanker. These incidents, however, may still require firefighters to wear standard personal protective equipment for extended periods. If it appears that the incident will exceed an hour in length, rehab operations should be considered.

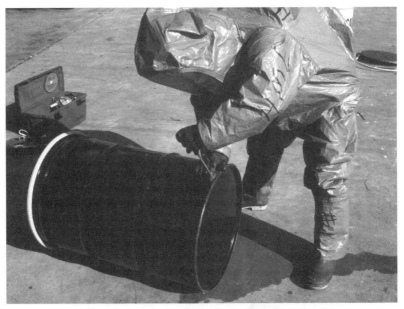

Figure 2-5 Protective clothing can shield emergency responders from the effects of hazardous materials but can also increase the likelihood of heat- and stress-related emergencies.

Weather Conditions

Up to this point, this chapter has focused on the types and durations of incidents as criteria in establishing rehab operations at an emergency scene. Another key element in making the determination is weather conditions at the time of the incident. In fact, in jurisdictions subject to extreme weather conditions, those conditions will often be the most important consideration in deciding whether or not to establish a rehab area. Most people automatically associate hot temperatures with the need for rehabbing emergency responders. Bear in mind, however, that extremely cold weather can be just as dangerous for emergency workers.

Hot-Weather Conditions

Even under the most "ideal" climatic conditions, fires, hazmat incidents, and rescue operations place a variety of thermal stresses on the responders operating at them. Emergency responders must frequently perform heavy physical labor in heated atmospheres (i.e., inside burning structures) while wearing bulky protective clothing. In those "ideal" conditions, when the responders have completed their assigned tasks, they can go to a safe area (such as rehab), remove their protective clothing, and cool down.

Unfortunately, not all emergency scene operations occur in such ideal climatic conditions. In some cases, ambient air temperatures are so high that firefighters may begin to suffer from heat stress even before beginning their assigned tasks. Once their tasks are completed, they are unable to cool down even after removing their protective clothing and equipment. Such conditions demand effective rehab operations, even at incidents that are smaller or shorter term than those described earlier in this chapter.

To better understand how hot weather affects the need for rehab, it is important to review some basic factors involving heat and the human body's response to it. In many cases, the actual air temperature at a given location, sometimes referred to as the *ambient temperature,* is not the sole factor in creating heat stress problems for emergency responders. The amount of heat stress that emergency responders are exposed to is actually a combination of three important factors (Figure 2-6):

- Ambient temperature
- Relative humidity
- Direct sunlight

In general, the amount of thermal stress that a person is exposed to is more accurately measured by combining the effects of the ambient temperature and *relative humidity* of the atmosphere. The relative humidity of an atmosphere is the amount of water vapor, or moisture, that is suspended in the air. Keep in mind that warm air can hold more moisture than colder air.

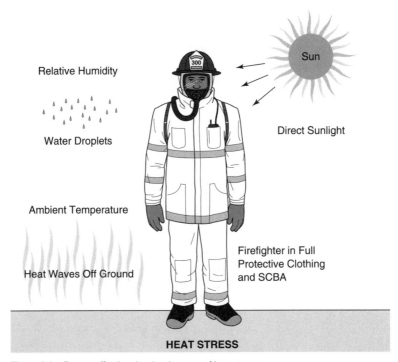

Figure 2-6   Factors affecting the development of heat stress.

Ambient air temperature and relative humidity can be factored together to create what is often referred to as the *heat stress index, heat index,* or *humiture.* Depending on the conditions, the reading on the heat stress index may indicate that the atmosphere feels warmer or cooler than the actual ambient temperature. For example, examine the figures contained in Table 2-1. Note that when the ambient temperature is 94°F (34°C) and the relative humidity is 10 percent, the heat stress index is 89°F (32°C). (Such a condition is common in places like Phoenix, Arizona.) On the other hand, when the ambient temperature is 94°F (34°C) and the relative humidity is 60 percent, the heat stress index is 111°F (44°C). (Such a condition is common in places such as Houston, Texas, or Baltimore, Maryland.)

In addition to ambient air temperature and relative humidity, the effects of direct sunlight on personnel should be considered. Remember that sun shining on the surfaces of objects produces radiated heat. If the responders are working in direct sunlight, factor in an additional 10°F (4°C) to the heat stress index reading.

Finally, when thinking about the heat stress index, think about the clothing that on-scene personnel are wearing. If emergency responders are required to wear heavy protective clothing, add 10°F (4°C) to the figure in the table.

Table 2-1 Heat Stress Index

Temperature, °F	Relative Humidity								
	10%	20%	30%	40%	50%	60%	70%	80%	90%
104	98	104	110	120	132				
102	97	101	108	117	125				
100	95	99	105	110	120	132			
98	93	97	101	106	110	125			
96	91	95	98	104	108	120	128		
94	89	93	95	100	105	111	122		
92	87	90	92	96	100	106	115	122	
90	85	88	90	92	96	100	106	114	122
88	82	86	87	89	93	95	100	106	115
86	80	84	85	87	90	92	96	100	109
84	78	81	83	85	86	89	91	95	99
82	77	79	80	81	84	86	89	91	95
80	75	77	78	79	81	83	85	86	89
78	72	75	77	78	79	80	81	83	85
76	70	72	75	76	77	77	77	78	79
74	68	70	73	74	75	75	75	76	77

Note: Add 10°F when protective clothing is worn and add 10°F when in direct sunlight.

There are no hard and fast rules stating the heat stress index level at which rehab operations should be established or increased in scale. A publication on rehab from the United States Fire Administration recommends that rehab operations be initiated whenever the heat stress index exceeds 90°F (32°C). In reality, each department is likely to have its own preferences on this matter based on the climatic conditions common in its jurisdiction. Jurisdictions where firefighters encounter higher temperatures on a regular basis may use a higher heat stress index level as a basis for altering standard rehab procedures than would jurisdictions that rarely experience higher heat stress indices. For example, the Anytown, Minnesota, Fire Department may choose to expand rehab operations when the heat stress index exceeds 90°F (32°C). That is because the index in Anytown rarely reaches that level and the department's responders are not accustomed (i.e., conditioned) to operating in those conditions. On the other hand, the Ship Channel, Texas, Fire Department may not initiate expanded rehab operations until the heat stress index exceeds 105°F (40°C) because its personnel are accustomed to operating in hot, humid conditions on a regular basis.

While there is no consensus on a particular heat stress index level that requires expanded rehab procedures, there are some commonly accepted parameters for the threat of injury related to elevated heat stress index conditions. Table 2-2 outlines these parameters. Individual departments may choose to consider these parameters when establishing SOPs for rehab. Incident Commanders should also keep these figures in mind when operating on an emergency scene.

Table 2-2   Injuries Associated with Heat Stress Index Conditions

Humiture, °F	Danger Category	Injury Threat
Below 60°	None	Little or no danger under normal circumstances
80° to 90°	Caution	Fatigue possible if exposure is prolonged and there is physical activity
90° to 105°	Extreme caution	Heat cramps and heat exhaustion possible if exposure is prolonged and there is physical activity
105° to 130°	Danger	Heat cramps and heat exhaustion likely and heat stroke possible if exposure is prolonged and there is physical activity
Above 130°	Extreme danger	Heat stroke imminent!

Many departments have SOPs that automatically go into effect when the heat stress index exceeds a predetermined temperature. Examples of these procedures include the following:

- An additional engine or truck company is dispatched on all full box assignments.
- An additional ambulance or EMS responder unit is dispatched on all working incidents.
- Specialized rehab equipment is automatically dispatched on calls where rehab would ordinarily be activated by a special call from the Incident Commander.
- Firefighters are required to report to rehab after expending one SCBA cylinder rather than the regular two cylinders.

Further information on operating in high heat stress conditions and the physical dangers associated with it is contained in chapter 4.

Cold-Weather Conditions

Often overlooked when determining the need for rehab operations are the effects of cold weather on responders who must operate in low-temperature conditions for long periods of time. Cold weather poses different rehab challenges to emergency responders than the warm-weather scenarios described above. The potential threat to the well-being of firefighters from them, however, is just as great.

Perhaps the issue of providing rehab to firefighters operating in cold-weather conditions is downplayed because of the heavy protective clothing that firefighters wear. While that protective clothing causes almost immediate heat-stress-related problems in hot weather, it does help shield wearers from the effects of cold temperatures in the winter. Because of the nature of fire-fighting and rescue operations, however, this benefit can eventually become a problem, even in severe cold weather.

One aspect of fire-fighting operations that increases the threat to firefighters in cold weather is the use of water. It is inevitable that firefighters will become wet at some point during operations. They may be splashed with water from hoses or puddles or exposed to large amounts of steam during interior fire-fighting operations. While protective clothing helps combat the effects of the cold when it is dry, once it or the firefighter wearing it becomes wet, its ability to protect the wearer from the cold is significantly reduced.

Also keep in mind that the human body burns more calories when temperatures are cold than when they are warm. This is because extra energy is required to maintain the body's normal core temperature in colder temperatures. As a result, emergency personnel may become hungry faster in cold weather than in warm weather. They may also require frequent breaks during periods of heavy exertion. These are issues that must not be overlooked when determining the need for rehab during winter operations.

While standard firefighter personal protective clothing provides sufficient protection from the cold in most climates, there are jurisdictions—Alaska, northern Canada, etc.—where the weather conditions are so severe that extra levels of cold-weather protection are required. In these areas, firefighters may have to wear additional insulated clothing beneath their normal protective clothing. They may also have to use protective clothing specially designed for extremely cold climates, for example, fire-fighting mittens as opposed to standard gloves. Wearing this additional protective gear increases the level of stress on firefighters.

In hot-weather conditions, the primary threat to the firefighter is a dramatic *rise* in the body's core temperature. This can cause a heat-related illness, such as heat stroke, that affects the entire body—in other words, a total, systemic illness. In cold conditions, the major problem is significantly different. A firefighter insufficiently protected against the cold may have his or her body's core temperature *lowered* to dangerous levels under extreme circumstances (Figure 2-7). This condition is commonly referred to as *hypothermia*. Like heat stroke, this is a total systemic illness. Cases of true hypothermia in emergency operations are fortunately rare. However, the risk of hypothermia must always be considered whenever personnel must operate in cold weather for excessive periods of time.

The most common cold-related injuries among emergency responders are localized cold injuries, commonly called *frostnip* or *frostbite*. These injuries occur when particular parts of the body are exposed to extreme cold for extended periods of time. Firefighters and other emergency responders frequently develop these localized cold injuries on the face, ears, hands, and feet.

Before learning how cold weather specifically affects the need for rehab, it is important to understand some basic principles related to cold temperatures and wind. Just as heat and humidity combine to increase the negative effects on a responder's body, so do cold temperatures and wind. Simply stated, any amount of wind in cold temperature conditions will make the climate feel even colder than it registers on a thermometer. For example, on a day when the actual temperature is 25°F (−4°C), a 20-miles-per-hour (32-kilometers-per-hour) wind will make the temperature feel like −3°F (−15°C). The combined effect of cold temperatures and wind is commonly referred to as the *wind chill factor, wind chill index,* or *wind chill temperature.* Table 2-3 contains wind chill factors for various temperatures and wind speeds.

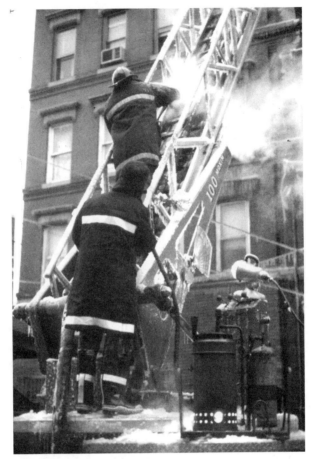

Figure 2-7 In cold-weather operations, a well-run rehab area can help reduce the risks of hypothermia.

A lower wind chill factor will not make water freeze faster or make machinery operate more sluggishly. For example, Table 2-3 shows that with an ambient temperature of 40°F (4°C) and a wind blowing at 30 miles per hour (48 kilometers per hour), the wind chill factor is 13°F (−10°C). While the personnel operating on a fire scene under these conditions feel much colder than they normally would at 40°F (4°C), the water being used on the scene will not freeze. For this to occur, the actual ambient temperature would have to be 32°F (0°C).

At these wind chill levels, hypothermia may develop in people exposed to weather conditions for excessively long periods, but this is not a common emergency services problem. The greatest dangers to emergency responders begin when the wind chill index drops below 25°F (−4°C). As the index drops from 25°F down to −75°F (−59°C), chances of personnel who are not properly protected suffering a cold injury increase. At the −75°F level, exposed flesh may freeze in as little as 30 seconds.

Table 2-3 Wind Chill Index

Wind Speed, mph	Temperature, °F												
	45	40	35	30	25	20	15	10	5	0	−5	−10	−15
5	43	37	32	27	22	16	11	6	0	−5	−10	−15	−21
10	34	28	22	16	10	3	−3	−9	−15	−22	−27	−34	−40
15	29	23	16	9	2	−5	−11	−18	−25	−31	−38	−45	−51
20	26	19	12	4	−3	−10	−17	−24	−31	−39	−46	−53	−60
25	23	16	8	1	−7	−15	−22	−29	−36	−44	−51	−59	−66
30	21	13	6	−2	−10	−18	−25	−33	−41	−49	−56	−64	−71
35	20	12	4	−4	−12	−20	−27	−35	−43	−52	−58	−67	−75
40	19	11	3	−5	−13	−21	−29	−37	−45	−53	−60	−69	−76
45	18	10	2	−6	−14	−22	−30	−38	−46	−54	−62	−70	−78

Wind Chill Temperature, °F	Danger
Above 25°	Little danger for properly clothed person
25° to −70°	Increasing danger; flesh may freeze
Below −75°	Great danger; flesh may freeze in 30 seconds

As with hot-weather conditions, individual jurisdictions determine at what wind chill index level rehab operations should be initiated or expanded. This determination is based on the normal weather conditions in the jurisdiction and the level of experience personnel have with cold-weather operations. No codes or standards dictate a specific level at which additional caution must be exercised. The USFA, however, recommends initiating rehab operations whenever the wind chill factor drops to 10°F (−12°C) or lower.

Incident Commanders operating in extremely cold conditions should think about some of the same tactical considerations that apply in hot-weather conditions. These include calling for additional companies and personnel, making sure appropriate rehab equipment is on the scene, and rotating personnel more frequently.

Postincident operations can also be adversely affected by extremely cold weather, in that hoses, ladders, and other equipment may become frozen in place. This means that considerable effort will be expended in freeing, retrieving, and stowing the equipment. Additional fresh, rested personnel may be needed to handle these tasks.

Further information on operating in cold-weather conditions and the physical dangers associated with it is contained in Chapter 4.

Other Situations Where Rehab May Be Necessary

The need for effective responder rehab operations is not limited to the "standard" types of emergency scenes or to the atmospheric conditions discussed so far in the chapter. A variety of other situations may necessitate the establishment of on-scene rehab operations. Although the scope of these possibilities is virtually endless, this section will examine some of the more common scenarios. Each jurisdiction should consider these types of activities when developing rehab policies for its agency.

Crime Scene/Standoffs

In recent years, the number of police operations of long duration has increased substantially. These operations include responses to bomb threats, hostage situations, incidents of civil unrest, and disturbed people posing threats to themselves and others. These operations can range in time from several hours to, in extreme cases, many weeks. Typically, many different agencies in addition to the police—fire, EMS, public works, for example—become involved in all or part of such operations.

These operations may take place in the environmentally challenging conditions discussed earlier in this chapter. Even if they don't, they generally involve large numbers of people, many of whom will be exposed to extreme mental stress, possibly for extended periods. Relief personnel must be available at these operations, and personnel relieved from forward operating positions must be monitored for any adverse physical or mental effects arising from the situation. In particular, the following personnel at crime scenes should be considered for mandatory, appropriate rehab treatment:

- Bomb squad members who have been operating in heavy protective clothing under extremely tense conditions for extended periods. The conditions, both physical and mental, that they experience will not be unlike those faced by hazmat technicians who have been operating in totally encapsulated suits for extended periods of time.
- Police tactical unit members who have been operating in forward positions for an extended period of time.
- Emergency personnel who have engaged in heavy physical labor during body recovery operations, the collection of evidence, or other scene activities.

Each jurisdiction should develop a policy indicating which agency will be responsible for responder rehab at a police operation. In some jurisdictions, each agency will handle its own members. A more effective approach is usually to pick a lead agency to perform the rehab functions. In most jurisdictions, the fire department or an EMS provider is the agency best suited to handle these functions.

Search Activities

Emergency response organizations are occasionally involved in extended search operations. These include situations such as the following:

- Large area searches for small children, the elderly, or mentally impaired individuals who have wandered away from their homes or care facilities.

- Urban search and rescue (USAR or US&R) incidents following natural or man-made disasters, such as structural collapses.
- Searches for climbers, hikers, or others involved in sports or recreation activities who become injured or lost in wildlands, caves, or similar settings.

Incidents such as these typically involve large numbers of responders, possibly from a variety of different agencies. Personnel participating in them usually do a lot of walking, climbing, lifting, and other intense physical activities. Often such incidents extend for many hours or days, and the responders need to maintain a sound physical and mental condition throughout the entire incident. Procedures must be in place to assure that personnel working at these incidents receive adequate nutrition, rehydration, and periods of rest.

Because these incidents often extend over a wide area, it may be necessary to have more than one Rehab group/sector. In some cases, it may be impractical to expect personnel to return to a designated rehab area. At such times, provisions must be made to bring food, drinks, and medical personnel to remote locations where personnel are operating. It may be necessary to use off-road vehicles or helicopters to reach some personnel.

Public Events

In addition to the emergency incidents covered so far, most jurisdictions must occasionally deal with planned events that require fire, EMS, and law-enforcement personnel to be in staged or standby positions for extended periods. In these cases, the personnel will need to be fed, provided liquids, and given adequate rest throughout the course of the events. Types of events that might require rehab for participating personnel include the following:

- Fairs, carnivals, or other festivals
- Auto races
- Parades
- Concerts
- Major sporting events
- Political rallies
- Large-scale religious ceremonies

With events like these, response agencies usually have the advantage of time in which to plan for rehab. Generally, an agency will have many weeks or months to prepare for an event. This will allow agency leaders to determine the number of personnel that will be needed on the scene, the duration that they will be there, and the types of rehab activities that will probably be necessary. In cases where sufficient manpower is available, it may be possible to completely relieve personnel of their assignments after a set period and send them home before they need to be rehabbed. In other cases, personnel may need to rotate through assignments, with time in rehab being a predetermined part of the duty rotation.

When planning for these events, agency leaders should anticipate a number of factors that will have a bearing on the nature or scope of required rehab activities. These include the following:

- The normal (and potentially adverse) weather conditions that can be expected for the time of year at which the event will be held.
- The ease of accessibility to the event in order to rotate personnel in and out. For example, traffic jams around a major speedway may prevent personnel from easily entering or exiting the area during the event.
- The level of physical activity that the personnel will be required to perform.
- The availability of appropriate areas and facilities to be used for rehab.

The persons responsible for managing the event at which responders will be operating must be advised of the agency's concerns and requirements for rehab. If the event organizers are unable to commit to providing all the resources required for taking appropriate care of responders, agency leaders should not commit their personnel to the event.

Training Activities

An area in which rehab is often required but too often overlooked is training activities for members of emergency agencies. Training activities frequently involve strenuous exercises that continue for extended periods of time. The same cautions and alertness for overexertion and responder well-being should be exercised at a training activity as would be used at an emergency scene.

Training facilities should be designed, or at least set up when used, with the ability to provide adequate participant rehab in mind. Shaded rest areas, climate-controlled structures, appropriate fluid replenishment stations, and other rehab needs should be included in plans for the training facility. All training classes or exercises should be designed so that rehab will be available to the participants for appropriate amounts of time at regular intervals.

Certainly, it is an excellent idea to set up a rehab operation on the training ground that mirrors that agency's policies for rehab operations at emergency scenes. This will allow trainees to understand how rehab works once they are out of the training atmosphere. It is also good practice for both new and experienced personnel in establishing rehab areas at emergency scenes.

REHAB WITHIN THE INCIDENT MANAGEMENT SYSTEM

One of the most basic tenets of running a safe and effective emergency scene is the use of a formal incident management system (IMS). All aspects of the emergency operation must work within the incident management system in order for it to be successful. Rehab operations are no exception to this principle. In order to understand how to organize and run an effective emergency incident rehabilitation area, it is necessary first to understand how rehab fits into the overall IMS picture.

The History of Incident Management Systems

Before 1970, no nationally or even regionally recognized incident management system existed. Individual fire departments typically had their own "systems" for running emergency scenes. In some cases, departments had systems that worked adequately for their needs at normal emergency operations. Those systems, however, often fell apart when other agencies attempted to assist in large-scale incidents. In point of fact, most emergency organizations had *no* formal incident management systems. Every incident was run a little differently (often depending on who was in charge on a given day). There was little overall consistency to incident scene operations.

This was the situation when a series of large wildland fires struck southern California in the early 1970s. These were some of the first "wildland/urban interface" fires, which have become increasingly common in recent years. This series of fires forced local, state, and federal fire protection agencies in the region to try to work together in order to extinguish the fires effectively. Before this time, most of these agencies had had little experience in working together on large incidents, and these new attempts were marred by disorganization.

Dissatisfaction with this disorganization led to the formation of an organization called FIRESCOPE (**Fire Re**sources in **S**outhern **C**alifornia **O**rganized to **P**rotect against **E**mergencies). Representatives of each of the organizations involved in the fires worked to develop a common management system that the agencies could use during any such events in the future, including fires, earthquakes, outbreaks of civil unrest, and other major incidents. The result of their labor was an incident management framework called the *Incident Command System* (ICS).

The agencies that helped develop ICS soon learned that it could be used with more than the occasional large, multiagency or multijurisdictional incident. All the agencies participating in FIRESCOPE soon adopted ICS into their daily operations.

Within a few years, ICS had been adopted for use in classes taught at the USFA's National Fire Academy in Emmitsburg, Maryland. Most federal agencies that responded to major emergencies also formally adopted ICS as their standard method of managing emergency incident operations. Soon, a significant number of local fire and emergency organizations throughout the United States had adopted ICS.

Nevertheless, the majority of emergency organizations still chose not to adopt ICS. There were a number of factors behind these refusals:

- Many emergency organizations are so bound by tradition that they have difficulty in implementing major new concepts within their organizations.
- There were no laws or standards that forced emergency organizations to adopt ICS or any other incident management system.
- Rivalry among emergency organizations in various regions of the country often stood in the way of one region's acceptance of new systems or technologies developed in other regions (the "left coast/right coast" mentality).
- There was a perception that ICS was solely designed for large-scale wildland fires and that it was not easily adaptable to the more routine types of incidents to which most agencies respond.

One of the agencies that did not quickly adopt ICS was the Phoenix, Arizona, Fire Department. While Phoenix department members recognized the need to develop better ways of handling emergency incidents, they felt that ICS was not the answer for their department. Eventually they developed a system that they called *Fire Ground Command* (FGC). This system was geared toward more commonly occurring types of incidents than wildland fires, in particular, those incidents that required fewer than 25 fire companies to control. FGC soon was adopted across North America by many agencies that had not previously embraced ICS.

There were two principal reasons for FGC's spread beyond the Phoenix city limits. First was *Fire Command*, a book on the system written by Phoenix Fire Chief Alan Brunacini and published by the NFPA. Second were the tireless efforts of Brunacini and other department members who traveled and taught hundreds, if not thousands, of seminars on the topic.

While FGC and ICS were similar in many respects, the two systems had enough differences to cause difficulties when agencies using the different systems tried to work together at emergency scenes. Leaders in the fire service saw these differences between the systems as potentially serious problems because emergency organizations were increasingly moving toward regional and national response capabilities. The Federal Emergency Management Agency's Urban Search and Rescue task force program is an excellent example of this move toward national response capabilities. This program has readily deployable rescue teams stationed all over the United States. If teams from different parts of the country were to assemble and then not be able to work together under a common incident management framework, serious problems might result. It became clear that someone needed to take the lead in merging the two most popular systems into a single system that all could agree on and use.

The organization that stepped up was the International Association of Fire Chiefs (IAFC). In 1990, IAFC formed a task group to look at merging ICS and FGC. Obviously, the principal players in the effort included representatives of FIRESCOPE and the Phoenix Fire Department. Many other fire service organizations and fire departments were represented as well. The task force decided early in its work that in order for the project to be successful, it needed to be independent of any one organization. Thus the IAFC task group evolved into a stand-alone organization that became known as the National Fire Service Incident Management System Consortium (Figure 2-8).

The consortium developed the merged system that is now known as the National Fire Service Incident Management System (IMS). In 1993, the consortium published the first document about IMS, describing how IMS applied to structure fires. Subsequent publications dealt with IMS and high-rise fires, emergency medical incidents, and urban search and rescue incidents. The consortium remains active today, preparing new publications on IMS applications in a variety of emergency response situations.

Most major national fire service organizations have now endorsed IMS as the system that should be used by all fire departments. As National Fire Academy

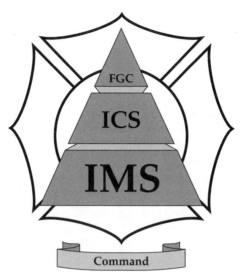

Figure 2-8 The logo of the National Fire Service Incident Management System Consortium.

courses are updated and rewritten, IMS is being integrated into them. Because IMS is likely to become the dominant management system in North America in the future, it will be the basis for incident management discussions in this book.

It should also be noted that today laws and standards require fire departments and other emergency service organizations to use formal incident management systems during emergency operations. OSHA regulations specifically require a system to be in place at any incident that involves hazardous material. NFPA 1500, *Standard of Fire Department Occupational Safety and Health Program,* requires all fire departments to have a formal incident management system in place and to use it during all emergency operations.

An Overview of IMS

The purpose of IMS is to provide for the systematic development of a complete, functional incident command organization. This command organization must work whether the incident involves a single agency or multiple agencies. Use of IMS increases the effectiveness of incident command and promotes enhanced firefighter safety.

IMS is designed to be the basic, everyday operating system for all incidents within an agency. When members of an agency are trained to use IMS on a daily basis, the transition to large and/or multiagency operations requires a minimum of adjustment.

The IMS organization builds from the ground up, with the management of all major functions initially being the responsibility of one or just a few persons.

Functional units are designed to handle the most important incident activities. As the incident grows in size and/or complexity, functional unit management is assigned to additional individuals in order to maintain a reasonable span of control and efficiency.

IMS is designed to assure that the jurisdictional authority of the involved agencies will not be compromised. Each agency having legal responsibility within its jurisdiction is assumed to have full command authority within its jurisdiction at all times. Assisting agencies will normally function under the direction of the Incident Commander appointed by the jurisdiction within which the incident occurs.

Establishing Command

The first emergency responder or unit to arrive at the scene should always assume command of the incident. The person in charge of the incident is referred to as the *Incident Commander.* The initial Incident Commander remains in command until command is transferred to another responder (usually of a higher rank) or until the incident is stabilized and terminated.

Formal establishment of command is not typically required on incidents that involve the response of a single company. Such incidents might include vehicle fires and EMS runs involving a single patient. In these cases, the company officer will simply acknowledge the company's arrival on the scene.

For incidents that require the commitment of multiple companies, the highest-ranking member of the first unit on the scene must formally establish and announce "Command." That person is charged with developing an incident management structure appropriate for the incident. This initial Incident Commander is also responsible for performing an initial evaluation of the conditions at the incident site (often referred to as a *size-up*), determining the initial actions that will be taken, and providing directions to other companies that are still en route to the scene. The results of the size-up should be reported to the dispatcher and other responding companies in a concise radio report. The radio report should include the following information:

- Unit designation of the unit arriving on the scene
- A brief description of the incident situation (building size, occupancy, hazmat release, multivehicle accident, etc.)
- Obvious conditions (working fire, hazmat spill, multiple patients, etc.)
- A brief description of the actions being taken
- The declaration of strategy, offensive or defensive (this applies to structure fires)
- Any obvious safety concerns
- Assumption, identification, and location of Command
- Request for, or release of, resources as required

The vast majority of incidents to which fire departments and other emergency agencies respond are handled by an Incident Commander and five or fewer companies. In these cases, all the company officers report directly to the Incident

Commander (Figure 2-9). It is generally assumed that the maximum effective span of control for any one supervisor (in this case the Incident Commander) is a ratio of 5 to 1. This means that a maximum of five persons should report directly to the Incident Commander. Therefore, if it becomes necessary to involve more than five companies on an incident, it will be necessary to organize multiple companies into larger subunits, with each subunit having one designated supervisor who reports to the Incident Commander.

There are two basic methods for organizing companies into subunits. The first method utilizes divisions and groups. *Divisions* are subunits that are assigned to a specific geographic location. For example, three engine companies assigned to the north side of a brushfire could be designated the "North Division." *Groups* are subunits that are assigned to perform a specific function. For example, two truck companies sent to cut a hole in the roof of a burning building might be designated the "Vent Group." In each of these cases, one of the company officers would be assigned to be in charge of all the companies in that subunit. That person would be known as the Division Supervisor or Group Supervisor. When rehab operations are established at small incidents, they are usually known as the Rehab Group.

The second method of organization employs the term *sector* to designate subunits that are given either geographic or functional assignments. Using the examples above, the subunits would be designated the North Sector or Vent Sector. The person in charge of these subunits would be the North Sector Supervisor or Vent Sector Supervisor. Rehab operations in these cases would be known as the Rehab Sector.

The National Fire Service Incident Management System Consortium recognizes both of the methods of designated subordinate IMS positions described

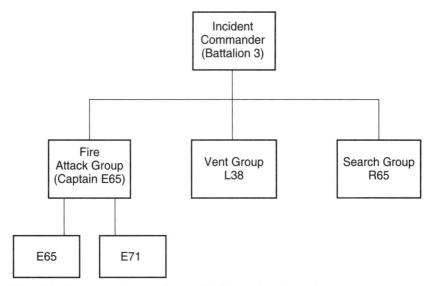

Figure 2-9   The command structure for a small incident such as a house fire.

previously. It recommends that local jurisdictions select the method that is most effective for them. The methods should not be mixed within a jurisdiction. Personnel, however, should be trained in both methods, in the event that a mutual-aid response requires them to interact with an agency that uses the other method.

Expanding the Incident

By utilizing divisions and groups or sectors, it is possible for up to 25 companies to operate on an emergency scene without anyone's span of control being exceeded (five companies reporting to each supervisor, five supervisors reporting to the Incident Commander). (See Figure 2-10.) If it becomes necessary to add more resources to an incident or if it would be more effective to break the original 25 companies into more focused work groups, the Incident Commander may choose to institute *branches* as the next level of the IMS structure.

Consider, for example, the case of a structure fire at an industrial facility that involves hazardous materials. There are also multiple casualties on the scene when emergency responders arrive. Rather than dividing the incident into various divisions, groups, or sectors, the Incident Commander may choose to establish branches to handle each major aspect of the operation. In this case, the branches might include a fire branch, a hazmat branch, and a medical branch (Figure 2-11). The person in charge of each branch is called the Branch Director (e.g., Medical Branch Director). On larger incidents, there may be multiple divisions, groups, or sectors within each branch.

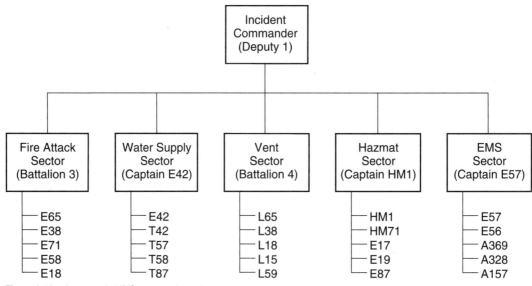

Figure 2-10 An expanded IMS command structure.

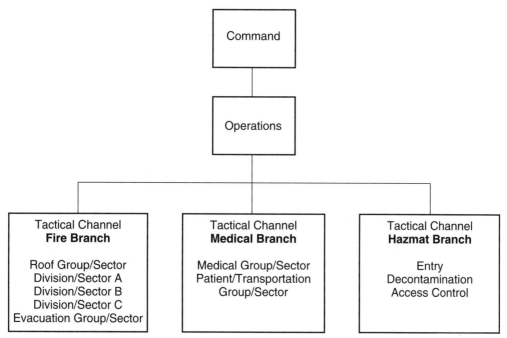

Figure 2-11   A basic IMS branch structure.

As the incident expands further, the Incident Commander has the option of activating one or more of four major *sections*, in addition to Command (Figure 2-12). These sections include:

- Operations
- Planning
- Logistics
- Finance/administration

Keep in mind that the Incident Commander is responsible for all the duties associated with each of these sections until that section is activated. If the Incident Commander chooses to activate only one or two of the sections at an incident, he or she remains responsible for the duties of the unactivated sections. Note that the functions of two or more sections should never be combined. The person in charge of a section is called the Section Chief (e.g., the Planning Section Chief).

Operations Section   The Operations Section is responsible for the direct management of all incident tactical activities, the tactical priorities, and the safety and welfare of the personnel working in the Operations Section (Figure 2-13). The Operations Section Chief uses the appropriate radio channel to communicate strategic and specific objectives to the branches, divisions/groups, or sectors.

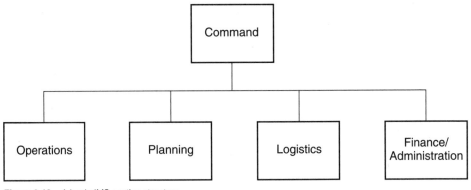

Figure 2-12 A basic IMS section structure.

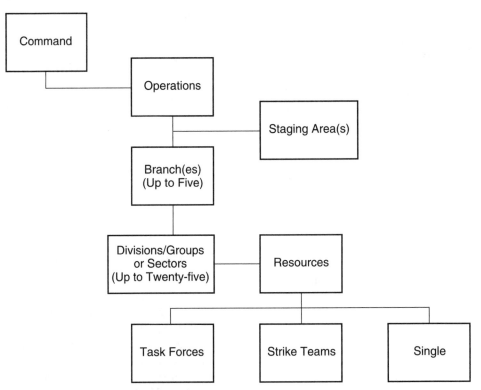

Figure 2-13 Structure of an operations section.

The Operations Section is most often implemented (staffed) as a span-of-control mechanism. When the number of branches, divisions/groups, or sectors exceeds the effective management capability of the Incident Commander, the Incident Commander may activate the Operations Section, thereby reducing the number of people reporting directly to him. The Operations Section Chief then assumes direct management of all tactical activities. Creation of this sector thus enables the Incident Commander to focus attention on management of the entire incident rather than diffusing it over a range of tactical activities.

The incident scene can quickly become congested with emergency equipment if that equipment isn't managed effectively. For major or complex operations, the Incident Commander should establish a central staging area early and place an officer in charge of Staging. A radio designation of "Staging" should be utilized. Once the Operations Section is activated, Staging reports to the Operations Section Chief. The Operations Section Chief may establish, move, and/or discontinue use of staging areas. All resources within the designated staging areas are under the direct control of the Operations Section Chief and should be immediately available.

Planning Section   The Planning Section is responsible for gathering, assimilating, analyzing, and processing information needed for effective decision making. Information management is a full-time task at large and complex incidents. The Planning Section serves as the Incident Commander's "clearinghouse" for information. The Planning Sector filters information from dozens of sources and provides the essential data to the Incident Commander's staff and to the Incident Commander. Critical information should be immediately forwarded to Command personnel (or whoever needs it). Information should also be used to make long-range plans. The Planning Section Chief's goal is to stay ahead of current events and to identify the need for resources before they are actually required.

There are provisions within IMS for the establishment of up to four units within the Planning Section if they become necessary (Figure 2-14). Each of these units, if activated, would be led by a Unit Leader. The Planning Section Chief is

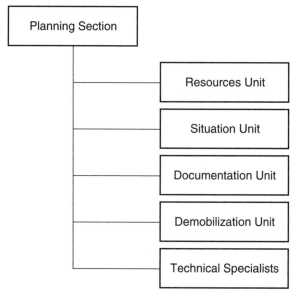

Figure 2-14   Structure of a planning section.

responsible for all duties of any unactivated units. The units within the Planning Section include:

- *Resources Unit.* This unit is responsible for all check-in activity, and for tracking the status of all personnel and equipment resources assigned to the incident. The unit is sometimes referred to as *Restat.*
- *Situation Unit.* This unit collects and processes information on the current situation, prepares situation displays and situation summaries, and develops maps and projections. In some cases, members of this unit may be required to do the reconnaissance necessary to obtain this information. This unit is sometimes called *Sitstat.*
- *Documentation Unit.* This unit documents the incident action plan, maintains all incident-related documentation, and provides duplication services. On some incidents it may be necessary for the Documentation Unit to work closely with the Finance/Administration Section.
- *Demobilization Unit.* On large, complex incidents, this unit will assist in assuring that an orderly, safe, and cost-effective movement of personnel will be made when those personnel are no longer required at the incident.

Any technical specialists that are required to handle the incident are also typically located under the Planning Section.

Logistics Section The Logistics Section is the support mechanism for the organization. Logistics provides services and support systems to all the organizational components involved in the incident including facilities, transportation, supplies, equipment maintenance, fueling, feeding, communications, and medical services, including rehab.

There are provisions within IMS for the establishment, if necessary, of up to six units under two branches within the Logistics Section (Figure 2-15). The Logistics

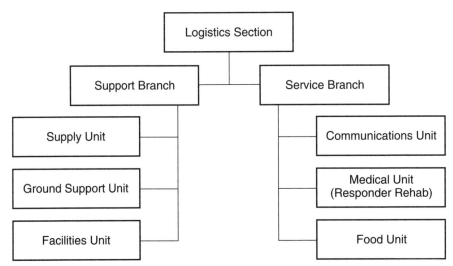

Figure 2-15 Structure of a logistics section.

Section Chief is responsible for all duties of any branch/unit that is not activated. The branches and units under the Logistics Section include:

- *Service Branch.* The Service Branch is supervised by the Service Branch Director.
  Communications Unit. This unit develops the incident communications plan, distributes and maintains all forms of communications equipment, and manages the incident communications center.
  Medical Unit. This unit develops the medical plan and provides first aid and light medical treatment for personnel assigned to the incident. It also develops the emergency medical transportation plan (ground and/or air) and prepares medical reports. The Medical Unit is *not* responsible for victims of the incident, only for emergency personnel assigned to work at the incident. Rehab operations fall under the responsibility of the Medical Unit. This is discussed in more detail later in this chapter.
  Food Unit. This unit is responsible for determining and supplying the nutritional and potable water requirements at all incident facilities and for active resources within the Operations Section. The unit may prepare menus and food, provide them through catering services, or use some combination of both methods.
- *Support Branch.* The Support Branch is supervised by the Support Branch Director.
  Supply Unit. The Supply Unit orders personnel, equipment, and supplies. This unit stores and maintains supplies and nonexpendable equipment. All orders are placed through this unit.
  Facilities Unit. This unit sets up and maintains whatever facilities may be required in support of the incident. It provides managers for the incident base and for additional camps. It also provides security support for the facilities and incident as required.
  Ground-Support Unit. This unit provides transportation and maintains and fuels vehicles assigned to the incident.

Finance/Administration Section   The Finance/Administration Section is established for incidents when the agencies that are involved have a specific need for financial services. Not all agencies will require the establishment of a separate Finance/Administration Section. In some cases where only one specific function is required—for example, cost analysis—that function could be performed by a Technical Specialist in the Planning Section.

There are provisions within IMS for the establishment of up to four units within the Finance/Administration Section if they become necessary (Figure 2-16). Each of these units, if activated, would be under the direction of a Unit Leader. The Finance/Administration Section Chief is responsible for all duties of any units that are not activated. The units within the Finance/Administration Section include:

- *Time Unit.* This unit assures that all time spent by personnel on an event or incident is recorded.
- *Procurement Unit.* This unit processes administrative paperwork associated with equipment rental and supply contracts. It is responsible for equipment time reporting.
- *Compensation/Claims Unit.* This unit handles two very important functions:
  Compensation is responsible for seeing that all documentation related to workers' compensation is completed correctly. Also, Compensation maintains files of injuries and/or illnesses associated with the incident.

Claims handles investigation of all claims involving damaged property associated with, or involved in, the incident.
- *Cost Unit.* This unit is responsible for collecting all cost information and providing cost estimates and cost savings recommendations.

Rehab's Place in IMS

As mentioned previously, in the fully expanded IMS the responsibility for rehab falls within the Medical Unit located in the Logistics Section. The Medical Unit is responsible for the overall well-being of responders who are on the scene. The Rehab group/sector is just one portion of the overall Medical Unit. In cases where there are no significant responder medical issues, rehab may be the only portion of the Medical Unit that is activated. In other cases, it will be necessary to integrate rehab functions into the other medical functions of the Medical Unit. Typically, this only occurs with very large-scale incidents.

The vast majority of incidents that most agencies deal with on a daily basis never evolve to the point where IMS sections are implemented. In fact, it is only on rare occasions that the need for branches ever becomes necessary. Therefore, we must examine rehab's place within the IMS system for the most common types of incidents.

In reality, it is not difficult to determine where rehab fits into the picture on small, routine incidents. As noted above, the Incident Commander is responsible for all portions of the IMS structure that are not specifically activated at a given incident (Figure 2-17). Thus, the Rehab group/sector will generally report directly to the Incident Commander. Even if the incident is divided into branches or if sections other than Logistics are implemented, the Rehab group/sector usually continues to report to the Incident Commander.

Some jurisdictions may choose to place rehab under the Operations Section if Logistics has not been activated (Figure 2-18). In these cases, the Rehab

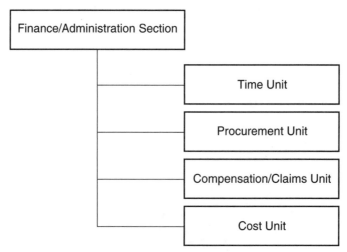

Figure 2-16 Structure of a finance/administration section.

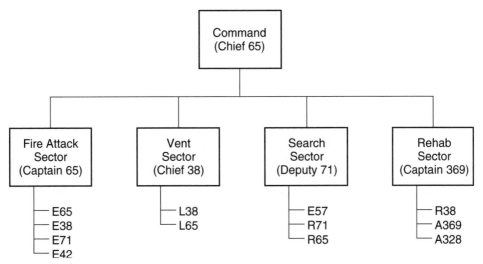

Figure 2-17   The position of Rehab in the command structure at a small incident.

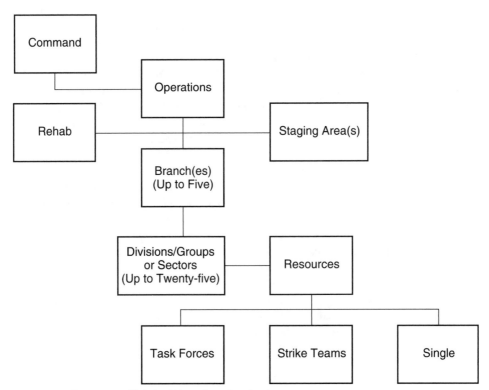

Figure 2-18   The position of Rehab within an Operations Section.

group/sector Supervisor, like the Staging Manager, reports to the Operations Section Chief. Technically, this arrangement is an incorrect use of IMS. However, some jurisdictions find that it works better for their needs.

REHAB'S ROLE IN THE PERSONNEL ACCOUNTABILITY SYSTEM

Keeping track of the movements and work locations of firefighters on an emergency scene is an extremely difficult task. It has been noted that UPS or Federal Express can better account for the whereabouts of a package anywhere in the world than the average Incident Commander can account for a firefighter on an emergency scene. Research by the NFPA has shown that firefighters who became disoriented or lost on the fireground accounted for 25 percent of non-stress-related firefighter deaths.

One of the keys to better tracking of personnel on the emergency scene is use of a proper IMS, such as the one described previously. Personnel who are working in groups with a supervisor who is responsible for them are less likely to get lost or go unaccounted for. Yet even fire departments that effectively used IMS have experienced serious firefighter injuries and deaths when firefighters became lost on a fireground. These situations tend to occur during interior fire attacks when fire conditions quickly worsen or a structural collapse occurs. A series of these types of incidents in the early- and mid-1980s led a number of fire departments to develop accountability systems to track personnel operating on an emergency scene.

An *accountability system* may be defined as a standard operating procedure used by an emergency response organization to track the locations and movements of responders on an emergency scene. Each department must develop its own accountability system that identifies and tracks all personnel working at an incident. The system should be standardized and used at every incident. All personnel must be familiar with the system and participate in it when operating at an emergency incident. The system must also account for those individuals who respond to the scene in vehicles other than fire department apparatus.

The use of an accountability system on the emergency scene is required by NFPA 1500 (1997 edition). Objective 6-3.1 of that document states, "The fire department shall establish written standard operating procedures for a personnel accountability system that is accordance with NFPA 1561, *Standard for Fire Department Incident Management Systems* and that provides for the tracking and inventory of all members operating on an emergency incident. The system shall provide a rapid accountability of all personnel at the incident scene."

Currently, the state of accountability systems is much the same as it was for incident management systems prior to the effort to combine ICS and FGC. A number of agencies have developed different accountability systems that have gained local or regional acceptance. No single model, however, has gained a major, national foothold. Some common systems that are used in the North American fire service include the Seattle PASSPORT system, the Phoenix Fireground Accountability system, and the Prince Georges County, Maryland, Personnel Accountability Tag (PAT) system.

It is not the purpose or intent of this book to advocate any one model over others. In general, most of the systems are fairly similar in nature. They employ some type of tag or token that specifically identifies a member and that is turned in when the member rides in position on a company or reports for duty at the scene of an emergency (Figure 2-19). The key to accurate accountability is the collection and control of these tags or tokens at the point of entry to the hazard area. The tags or tokens should then by organized in a way that instantly identifies where firefighters are working and which are in and which are out of the hazard area. Typically, the lower end of the system starts with all the members of a company placing their identifiers in a common location on the apparatus. As companies are grouped together on an emergency scene, an accountability officer is assigned to monitor the personnel of all the companies assigned to that division, group, or sector (Figure 2-20). When a company leaves its assigned area as a crew, its members pick up their identifiers from the accountability officer and bring them to their next destination. For example, suppose a crew that was making an interior attack in the front of a structure is ordered to withdraw and proceed to the rear of the structure to protect exposures. As the crew leaves the front of the building, its members pick up their identifiers from the front accountability officer and give them to the rear accountability officer when they arrive in that area.

Accountability in Rehab

Obviously, if the goal of the accountability system is to track personnel no matter where they are on the emergency scene, that includes tracking their presence in the

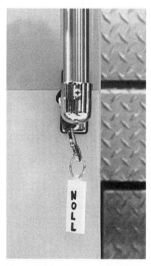

Figure 2-19 An accountability tag.

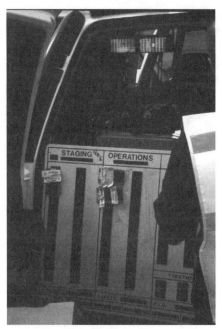

Figure 2-20   Accountability tags grouped on a board in the Command area.

Rehab group/sector. When a company or crew is removed from the action and sent to Rehab, its members should pick up their identifiers and present them to the Rehab Supervisor or Rehab accountability officer when they reach Rehab. The Rehab Supervisor should then place the identifiers in a prominent, predetermined location and record the entry of company/crew members on a check-in/check-out log sheet. This allows Rehab personnel to keep track of the companies/crews that are in their area. If a structural collapse or other serious problem develops, the Incident Commander will be able to determine quickly that the companies in Rehab are accounted for.

Once the company/crew has been sufficiently rehabbed and is ready as a group to be reassigned, command should be notified of the group's ready status. When the group receives its next assignment, its members should retrieve their identifiers from the Rehab Supervisor and take them along to their next assignment. The Rehab Supervisor should also note on the log sheet the time that company/crew members are checking out. If the company/crew is returning to service, the members will simply replace the identifiers on their apparatus when they are back in service.

The Rehab Supervisor should not return accountability identifiers to the company or crew until all its members are fit for duty. If one member of the crew is not fit for duty or is transported to a medical facility, that person's identifier should be removed from the rest of the group's, and it should be forwarded to the Incident Commander. The rest of the crew, if sufficient in number, may then be reassigned.

SUGGESTED READINGS

Brunacini, Alan. *Fire Command.* Quincy, MA: National Fire Protection Association, 1985.

Christen, Hank, and Maniscalco, Paul M. *The EMS Incident Management System.* Upper Saddle River, NJ: Brady/Prentice Hall, 1998.

Fire Protection Publications. *Incident Command System.* Stillwater, OK: Fire Protection Publications, 1983.

Fire Protection Publications. *Model Procedures Guide for High-Rise Fire Fighting.* Stillwater, OK: Fire Protection Publications, 1996.

Fire Protection Publications. *Model Procedures Guide for Structural Fire Fighting.* Stillwater, OK: Fire Protection Publications, 1993.

Fire Protection Publications. *Model Procedures Guide for Emergency Medical Incidents.* Stillwater, OK: Fire Protection Publications, 1996.

Fire Protection Publications. *Model Procedures Guide for Structural Collapse and Urban Search and Rescue.* Stillwater, OK: Fire Protection Publications, 1998.

United States Fire Administration. *Emergency Incident Rehabilitation.* Emmitsburg, MD: United States Fire Administration.

3

ESTABLISHING AND MANAGING A REHAB AREA

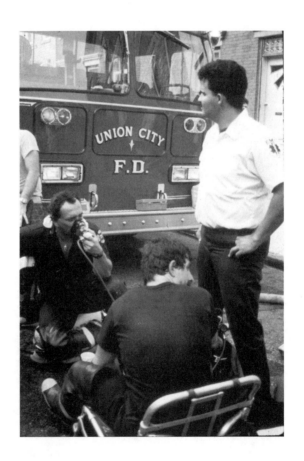

Once the Incident Commander has determined that it is necessary to establish rehab operations at an incident, responsibility for those operations will usually be transferred to another member of the organization who is on the scene of the incident. The person who accepts the responsibility for operating the Rehab group/sector must know how to select an appropriate location, obtain the necessary resources, and manage the rehab operation in an effective manner. This chapter discusses these important considerations in the establishment and management of the Rehab group/sector.

CHOOSING A REHAB AREA

Once the need for a Rehab group/sector has been determined, one of the most important decisions that must be made, and one that must be made almost immediately, is where to locate the rehab operations. Most organizations will have guidelines for the location of the rehab area in their standard operating procedures. All command staff and any other members of the organization who may be responsible for making the site selection must be familiar with these SOPs.

Making a good initial choice for the site of the Rehab group/sector is vital, because trying to relocate rehab operations in the middle of an emergency incident creates delay and confusion both for rehab personnel and for the crews who need rehab services. Therefore, one of the first things that must be understood when choosing a rehab area location is exactly who makes the decision. Fire department SOPs usually either specify the criteria for the decision or delegate the responsibility to the Incident Commander or the rehab unit leader.

- *Departmental SOPs.* In some cases, departmental SOPs provide very specific requirements for where the rehab area will be located. This is particularly true for agencies that operate specialized apparatus dedicated solely to providing rehab service. (These apparatus will be discussed later in this chapter.) The SOPs may dictate that rehab apparatus be located as close to Command as possible. If the SOPs do provide specific instructions on rehab location, they should always be followed as closely as possible. This is because on-scene personnel will have expectations of where to find rehab when they need it. If it becomes necessary to deviate from the SOPs, all personnel on the scene should be notified of the new location for the rehab area.
- *The Incident Commander.* In some jurisdictions, the Incident Commander determines the location for rehab. The Incident Commander will select a site based on the characteristics of both the scene and the incident. Factors that might influence the selection of the rehab area include the possibility of positioning close to the portion of the scene where the most intensive work is being performed; the availability of a location upwind of any hazardous gases or smoke; and the potential size of the incident—could it grow and force relocation of the rehab area? If the Incident Commander does select the site, information about the choice should be provided immediately to the person or company responsible for organizing and managing the site, as well as to all other personnel operating on the scene.
- *The Rehab Unit Leader.* Some agencies allow the Rehab Unit Leader to select the site for the rehab area. In these cases, the Incident Commander usually determines

the need for rehab operations and then appoints a person or company to initiate the rehab operations and choose the site. If this is the case, the Rehab Unit Leader should notify Command of the rehab site as soon as it is determined. This information should also be passed on to all personnel operating on the scene. Many jurisdictions prefer leaving the siting decision with the Rehab Unit Leader because that person can focus more intently on the decision than the Incident Commander, who has many other elements of the incident to consider.

Locating the Rehab Area

There are two basic schools of thought about what constitutes an ideal location for the rehab area. In some jurisdictions, it is felt that the best location is as close to Command as possible. In other jurisdictions, the goal is to place rehab in a location as far from incident operations as is reasonably possible. There are solid supporting reasons for each approach.

Those who choose to place rehab close to Command do so in order to allow the Incident Commander to keep track more easily of how many personnel are in rehab at any given time (Figure 3-1). This also makes it easier to anticipate when rehabbing companies will become available and ready for a new assignment. Another advantage of placing rehab operations near the command post is that doing so allows support vehicles to cluster at one location, thus making most efficient use of the equipment. For example, a single power and floodlight unit will be able to power and illuminate both the rehab and command areas. This is especially important in jurisdictions with limited resources.

Jurisdictions that choose to locate rehab operations away from the incident do so for several reasons. Some people feel that the farther the responders are from the incident, the more easily they will be able to rest and relax. In addition, there will be less of a tendency for responders to want to "jump back into the battle" before they are physically or emotionally ready. A more distant siting may also reduce the temptation for some command officers to place companies back into service too soon. Such a temptation can be hard to resist when the Incident Commander has a long list of things that need to be done and a couple of dozen firefighters are visible sitting in the rehab area.

Rehab Area Site Characteristics

Once this basic siting decision—close to or removed from the incident—is made, the next step in establishing a rehab area is choosing a specific location. The key rehab consideration is picking a location that truly allows firefighters and rescue personnel to get physical and psychological rest. However, departmental SOPs and other incident-related factors will have a bearing on the selection of the exact site.

If a jurisdiction chooses to locate rehab close to Command, there will be little leeway in the selection of the rehab site. In many cases, jurisdictions have a designated rehab vehicle that will be positioned near the command vehicle(s). This will

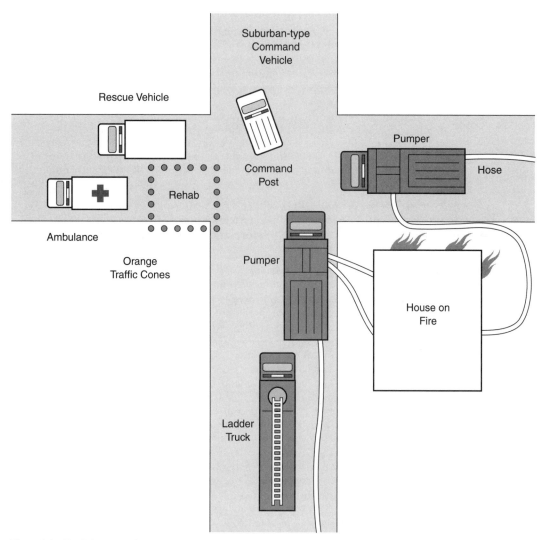

Figure 3-1   The Rehab group/sector should be located near the Command Post.

pretty much lock in the rehab site at that point. Even in these circumstances, the Rehab Unit Leader should nevertheless try to select a location that takes into consideration as many of the site characteristics listed below as possible.

If the Rehab Unit Leader is not locked into placing rehab adjacent to Command, the area immediately surrounding the scene may be searched for the best rehab location. During that search, the Rehab Unit Leader should keep the following considerations in mind:

- *The estimated number of responders who will need to be rehabbed.* On a small incident with a few companies on the scene, probably only one company will need to be rehabbed at a time. This level of rehab can be accomplished in the climate-controlled cab of an apparatus, the back of an ambulance, or a similar location. Larger numbers of responders mean that a larger location will be required.

- *The climatic conditions at the time of the incident.* If the weather is mild and dry, it may not be necessary to select a location that shelters the responders. If it is excessively hot or cold or if any type of precipitation is falling, however, it will be necessary to seek a site that provides shelter.
- *The duration of the incident.* If the incident is going to last for the better part of a day or longer, it may be desirable to locate a building in which rehab may be housed. Keep in mind, however, that if the building is a place of business, tying it up for a long time could be disruptive (and harmful) to the owner/occupant. Try to select a location that does not have an adverse effect on members of the general public.

Bearing these issues in mind, the Rehab Unit Leader can then set out to pick the site for rehab. The following list contains some of the more important site characteristics that must be considered before making a final selection:

- *The site should be outside, uphill, and upwind of the operational hazard area or "hot zone."* This allows personnel to remove their turnout gear and SCBAs safely.
- *The site should permit prompt reentry into emergency operations when personnel have completed rehabilitation.* The rehab area should not be so remote that the responders have to expend excessive energy traveling back to the scene.
- *The site should provide protection from environmental extremes, if necessary.* Locations such as a shaded, cool area in hot weather and a warm, dry, wind-protected area during cold-weather operations are preferred.
- *The site should be large enough to accommodate all those who may need rehabilitation.* Remember when laying out the site that crews in rehabilitation will need room to sit or lie down. In addition, there are accountability, medical, and rehydration functions that must be carried out in a rehab area. Space for these functions must be planned for, particularly on larger incidents.
- *The site should be free of vehicle exhaust.* If running vehicles are a part of the rehab operation, they should be positioned so that their exhausts discharge downwind of rehabbing personnel.
- *The site should be as quiet as possible.* Noise can have negative effects on efforts at stress reduction. When possible, locate the rehab area away from loud vehicles, equipment, and other sources of loud noise.
- *The site should restrict access by the media.* Tired, hungry, thirsty, stressed personnel generally do not make the best media spokespersons. If necessary, instruct law-enforcement personnel assigned to the rehab area to turn away any members of the media who try to interfere with personnel in rehab.
- *The site should provide access to SCBA replenishment/refill.* Allow room for apparatus that can carry large numbers of spare SCBA cylinders or that have cascade systems or breathing air compressors to be located at the rehab area.
- *The site should have easy entrance and exit routes for ambulances.* This will be important in the event that it becomes necessary to transport responders to the hospital for further evaluation and treatment.
- *The site should have a supply of running and drinkable water.* This simplifies ongoing rehydration operations. It also enables rehab crews to set up a cooling water spray in hot conditions.

- *It is helpful if rest room facilities are a part of the rehab area or are in close proximity to it.*
- *If the incident involves the recovery of fatalities, the rehab site should be out of view of the work area.* This will make it easier for rehabbing personnel to relax and take their minds off the difficult conditions they are operating under.

Once the site is selected, its location should be made known to all incident participants. In large-scale incidents, more than one Rehab group/sector may be needed. If more than one area is established, rehab personnel at each site must keep accurate logs of the entries and exits of crews in order to assure proper fireground accountability. If the departments involved use a formal accountability system (such as passports), make sure all standard procedures for collecting and returning the identifiers are followed.

REHAB APPARATUS AND EQUIPMENT

In order to establish an effective rehab operation, it will be necessary to have the appropriate apparatus and equipment in place. The following section describes various types of apparatus and equipment that might be employed during a rehab operation. Not all incidents will require all the apparatus or equipment listed here. In some jurisdictions some of this apparatus or equipment may not even be available. However, jurisdictional or departmental leaders may use the information in this section to assess their level of "rehab readiness" and to determine types of apparatus or equipment they may wish to work into future plans.

Apparatus at the Rehab Area

Listed below are some of the apparatus commonly found at rehab areas and descriptions of the roles they play in rehab operations.

Pumpers and Aerial Apparatus

Standard pumpers and aerial apparatus (engine and truck companies) may play limited roles at the rehab area (Figure 3-2). As mentioned above, the climate-controlled cabs of these apparatus may be used as shelter and rest areas on smaller incidents. Many jurisdictions routinely deliver emergency medical services from engine and truck companies. In those cases, the apparatus may have EMS supplies that can assist rehab operations as well.

If engine or truck companies are assigned to staff rehab areas and their apparatus are not going to be used for shelter, the apparatus should be parked out of the way with the engines turned off. Doing this will eliminate any chance of vehicle exhaust and noise becoming a problem in the rehab area. The firefighters assigned to these companies should take all EMS and other equipment that might be useful to the rehab operation with them when they leave the apparatus.

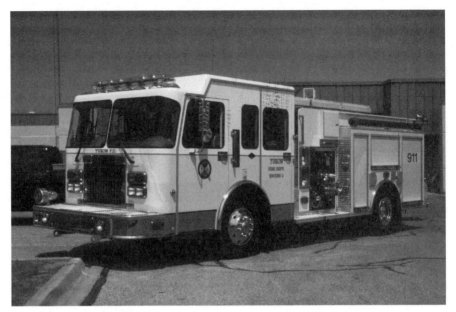

Figure 3-2   A pumper, especially one with a large crew cab, can be useful in rehab operations.

Rescue/Squad Apparatus

It is quite common for rescue or squad apparatus to be assigned to rehab operations (Figure 3-3). There are a number of reasons for this:

- In many jurisdictions, the rehab equipment is carried on the rescue vehicle. This is made possible by the large amount of storage space on the vehicle.
- Many rescue vehicles have large, climate-controlled bodies and cabs. They may be used to shelter anywhere from four to twelve or more responders, depending on the size of the vehicle.
- Rescue vehicles are often equipped with large electric generators and numerous floodlights. They can help provide electrical energy to the rehab area (and to the command post if they are co-located) as well as proper lighting for nighttime operations. In some jurisdictions, rescue vehicles also carry basic rehab equipment and supplies that can be used to initiate rehab operations.
- Many rescue vehicles carry spare SCBA cylinders or are equipped with cascade systems or breathing air compressors to refill expended cylinders.
- Some jurisdictions carry mass-casualty incident supplies on rescue apparatus. These extra supplies are also helpful to rehab operations.

In many jurisdictions, firefighters assigned to rescue companies also have more advanced emergency medical training than do other members of the department. This makes rescue company members better suited to handle the medical aspects of the rehab operation.

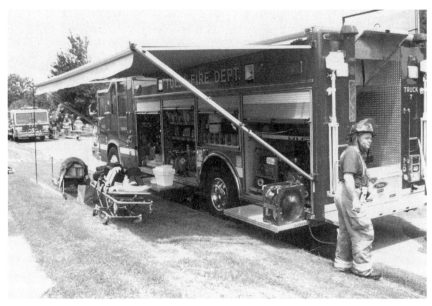

Figure 3-3   Rescue apparatus is commonly assigned to rehab operations.

EMS Vehicles

Because assuring the appropriate medical evaluation, treatment, and monitoring of personnel is one of the primary purposes of rehab, it is only natural that EMS vehicles and crews will have prominent places in the rehab area. Two basic types of EMS vehicles are used in rehab operations, transport and nontransport vehicles.

The more common term for an EMS transport vehicle is an ambulance. Ambulances will be located at the rehab area for one or more of four primary reasons:

- Their crews are assigned to staff the rehab area.
- They may be used to transport responders who need a greater level of care to a medical facility.
- Their EMS supplies are needed in the rehab area.
- They may be used for shelter during inclement weather.

Ambulances that are parked in or near the rehab area should be positioned so that they can be loaded rapidly and exit the area quickly should a responder need to be transported. Other vehicles in and around the rehab area should be parked to assure that entrance and exit routes for ambulances are not blocked.

Nontransport EMS vehicles are special vehicles that are used by EMTs, paramedics, or EMS supervisors to respond quickly to scenes and to begin treatment of victims until an ambulance can arrive and provide transport to a hospital

(Figure 3-4). These vehicles may carry a variety of equipment that could be useful in the rehab area. In some jurisdictions, it is common to appoint an EMS supervisor or lead paramedic as the Rehab Unit Leader. In such cases, these personnel will want their own vehicle close by so they can operate out of it in their supervisory capacity.

Mobile Air-Supply Units

Many fire departments have separate apparatus whose function is to refill or replace exhausted SCBA cylinders at emergency scenes. Such units may carry either a large number of air cylinders for replacement or a single or multiple cascade system or a breathing air compressor for refilling SCBA and cascade cylinders (Figure 3-5). Tools and parts are carried on the apparatus to make field repairs, adjustments, and replacements to damaged SCBA. The types of vehicles used for this function range from pickup trucks with trailers to larger vans or custom-designed apparatus. These units may be combined with other operations such as floodlight apparatus and rescue.

Mobile air-supply units are parked at the rehab area so that firefighters who are in rehab may have their SCBA cylinders refilled before returning to service. Whether the rehabbing firefighters receive another on-scene assignment or are told to return to quarters, their SCBAs should be refilled before they leave rehab. Jurisdictions that routinely send mobile air-supply units on structure fires and

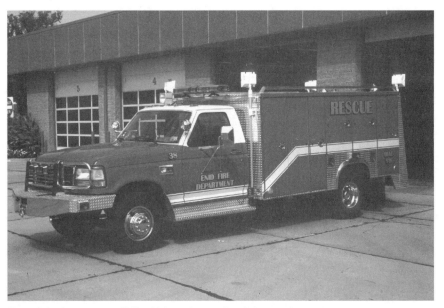

Figure 3-4   A nontransport EMS vehicle can be used in rehab operations.

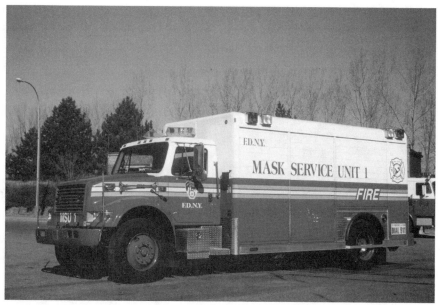

Figure 3-5   A mobile air-supply unit.

hazmat incidents commonly carry some rehab supplies on the unit. They may also carry items such as water jugs and cups for fluid replenishment.

Power and Light Units

Some fire departments have special apparatus to furnish lights and power at the scene of an incident (Figure 3-6). Large-capacity generators are used to power electric tools, provide standby power to buildings, and light the emergency scene. Auxiliary motors power the trailer- or truck-mounted generators. Banks of flood-lights and telescoping towers are provided, as well as an ample supply of extension cords, adapters, and portable lights. In many cases, power and light units are combined with air-supply units onto one vehicle. These are called air/power/light units.

Power and light units are helpful at the rehab scene during night operations. Departments that choose to locate rehab close to the command post often do so because the power and light unit can provide electric power to both areas.

Canteen Units

Canteen units are special vehicles whose primary function is to provide food and drinks to emergency responders at extended operations. Some fire departments operate their own canteen units. In most jurisdictions, however, non-fire department organizations operate the canteen units. Such organizations include the Red Cross, Salvation Army, fire buff organizations, fire department Ladies' Auxiliaries,

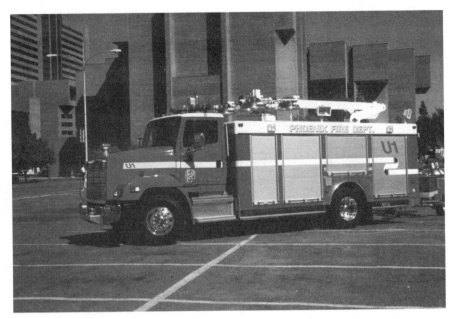

Figure 3-6   A power and light unit.

community service clubs (Lions, Elks, etc.), and other independent volunteer relief organizations.

Canteen units are mobile kitchens with a variety of capabilities and equipment. They may be equipped with ranges, fry griddles, ovens, microwave ovens, freezers/refrigerators, sinks and water tanks, large hot- and cold-drink dispensing equipment, and trash receptacles. Most have on-board electric generators for independent operation, as well as the ability to use power from an external source.

Emergency response organization leaders should encourage non-fire department canteen providers to offer foods and beverages that meet departmental policies for rehab operations. Responders on the scene might appreciate greasy hamburgers and soda pop, but fruit and fluid replacement drinks are more appropriate. Chapter 5 contains more information on appropriate food and drinks.

Rehab Vehicles

Some jurisdictions have vehicles that are designed and equipped specifically to perform rehab functions. These vehicles may be refurbished ambulances or rescue-type vehicles or custom-designed rehab units (Figure 3-7). Some rehab vehicles are intended simply to carry rehab equipment to the scene. Others are designed to provide shelter and be a physical part of the rehab area. They may contain rest/seating areas, toilets, medical evaluation areas, and limited refreshment serving areas.

The types of portable equipment carried on rehab vehicles will vary depending on the wishes and capabilities of the jurisdiction maintaining the vehicle.

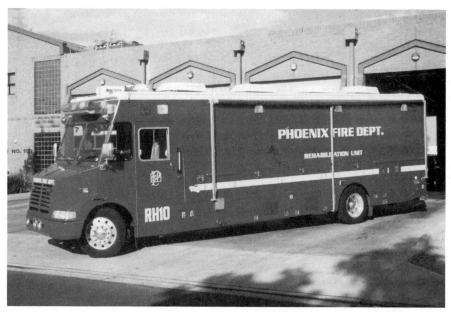

Figure 3-7   Some jurisdictions use vehicles specifically designed for rehab operations.

The equipment may include any or all things that are described in the section on rehab equipment.

Buses

Many jurisdictions that cannot afford dedicated rehab vehicles rely on buses from outside agencies for shelter during rehab operations. City transit and airport or rental-car shuttle buses work best for these applications. School buses can also be used. Whatever types of buses are used, they should be air-conditioned in warm-weather operations or heated for cold-weather operations. Emergency response agencies should have working agreements in place with bus providers. In some jurisdictions, the dispatch center automatically notifies the bus provider when an incident occurs in certain weather conditions. The bus provider then automatically dispatches a bus to the scene.

Rehab Equipment

A wide variety of equipment may be used in rehab operations. Not every agency will have all the types of equipment discussed here. Keep in mind also that the types of supplies or equipment that may be needed to establish a rehab area are not limited to the items discussed here. The items in this section represent the most common types of equipment that fire departments and other emergency organizations carry to the scene for rehab operations. Note that, in addition to this equipment, emergency medical equipment and supplies are vital for rehab operations. That medical material is discussed Chapter 4.

Portable Shelters

Portable shelters are used to protect responders from inclement weather and to shield them from sunlight during hot weather. Types of portable shelters commonly used for rehab operations include the following:

- Large tents
- Pop-up canopies or pavilions
- Air-inflated structures
- Foldout awnings that can be attached to the sides of rehab, rescue, or canteen vehicles (Figure 3-8)

Portable shelters intended for use at emergency scenes should be easily deployed by a minimum of personnel. During windy weather, it may be necessary to secure the shelters to the ground or to other fixed objects. In excessively windy conditions, it may not be possible to erect portable shelters.

Fans/Blowers

Fans and blowers may be used to assist in cooling responders who are resting in the shade. The moving air the fans and blowers provide will help bring down body temperatures more rapidly. Only electrically powered fans should be used for this function. Gas-powered blowers would vent their exhausts into the rehab area.

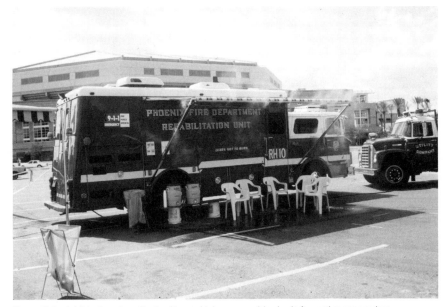

Figure 3-8   A foldout awning attached to a vehicle can provide shade for resting responders.

Two types of electric fans are commonly used for rehab functions. The first type is the common box fan that can be purchased in any hardware, appliance, or department store. The other commonly used type is the fire department smoke ejector. Because many fire departments have switched to gas-powered blowers for ventilation operations in recent years, many old, electric-powered smoke ejectors have found a second life in performing rehab functions. If possible, the smoke ejector should be fitted with an expandable air duct. This allows the smoke ejector to be located away from the rehab site while still supplying fresh air. Doing this will help reduce noise in rehab. Electric fans in the rehab area will require a source of electric power. Most commonly, power will be provided by an electric generator on a piece of fire apparatus.

Tarps and Blankets

Tarps and blankets have a variety of uses in the rehab area. They may be spread on the ground so equipment can be set down on them. In dirty or wet locations, they may provide more comfortable resting surfaces for rehabbing personnel. They may be used to construct lean-tos or sunscreens if portable shelters are not available. In cold weather, personnel may use warmed blankets to return their body temperatures to normal levels more quickly.

Tarps and blankets are commonly found on rescue vehicles, truck companies, ambulances, and rehab vehicles. Almost any type of tarps or blankets will work for the uses described above.

Portable Heaters

Portable heaters may be needed in jurisdictions that operate in colder climates. The heaters are placed in the rehab area to provide some increased comfort to resting firefighters. The two most common types of portable heaters used in rehab areas are electric and LPG-fired models. The portable electric heaters may be similar to those used in home or office settings. Obviously, some source of electric power in the rehab area will be necessary to operate these units.

LPG-fired portable heaters are also often referred to as *bullet heaters* or *salamanders* and are commonly used in the construction industry (Figure 3-9). They are fueled by small LPG cylinders connected to the heaters by flexible hoses. Keep in mind that these units will produce carbon monoxide as they operate. They should only be used in extremely well-vented areas. Some jurisdictions may wish to place carbon monoxide detection equipment in an area where gas-fired heaters are being used to assure that CO levels remain acceptable.

Make sure that all heaters are placed a safe distance from any combustible materials when used. The heaters should be inspected on a regular basis to assure that they are in safe operating condition.

Dry Clothing/Personal Protective Equipment

Some agencies keep supplies of dry clothing and personal protective equipment that may be placed in rehab areas for responders to change into as the need arises. Such

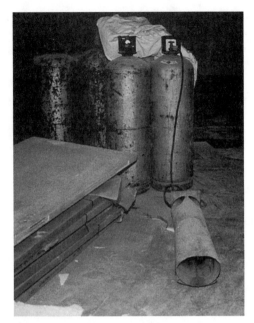

Figure 3-9   An LPG-fired portable heater.

a practice is particularly helpful in cold-weather operations, when the responders have become wet. This clothing and equipment is most commonly carried on rehab vehicles, rescue trucks, and special service vehicles. Agencies that provide extra clothing and protective gear should have established procedures for collecting the items after an incident. After an incident, the items should be washed and inspected before they are again placed on the apparatus.

For large-scale events, it may be necessary to bring extra clothing and protective equipment from departmental storage locations to the scene. Once again, departments should have procedures to account for and recover any items that are placed in service.

Lighting and Electric Generation Equipment

It is almost always necessary to use electrical equipment in the rehab area. If a ground shore source of electric power is not available, the electricity must be generated at the scene. A number of different types of electric generation equipment may be used to supply power to rehab areas.

Inverters (alternators) are used on some emergency vehicles to generate limited amounts of power. The inverter is a step-up transformer that converts the vehicle's 12- or 24-volt direct current into 110- or 220-volt alternating current. Advantages of inverters are their fuel efficiency and their low or nonexistent noise levels during operation. Disadvantages include small capacities and limited mobility from the vehicle. These units are generally capable of providing up to approximately 1,500 watts (1.5 kilowatts) of electric power. They are most commonly used to power vehicle-mounted floodlights.

Generators are the most common power sources used for emergency services. They can be portable or fixed to apparatus (Figure 3-10). Portable generators are powered by small gasoline or diesel engines and generally have 110- and/or 220-volt capacities. They can be operated in the compartments of apparatus, or they can be carried to remote locations. Most portable generators are designed so that they may be carried by one or two people. They are extremely useful when electric power is needed in areas not accessible to the vehicle-mounted systems. Portable generators are designed with a variety of power capabilities, with 5,000 watts (5 kilowatts) being the largest.

Vehicle-mounted generators usually have a larger power production capability than portable units. Vehicle-mounted generators can be powered by gasoline, diesel, or propane engines or by hydraulic or power takeoff systems. Fixed floodlights are usually wired directly to these units through switches, and outlets are also provided for other equipment. These power plants generally have 110- and 220-volt capabilities; capacities up to 12,000 watts (12 kilowatts) are common on pumpers. Rescue vehicles and air, power, and light apparatus commonly have larger generators. Capacities of up to 50,000 watts (50 kilowatts) are common. Mounted generators, particularly those powered by separate engines, are noisy, and conversation is difficult near them.

Lighting equipment may also be needed to illuminate the rehab area during nighttime operations. Lighting equipment can be divided into two categories: fixed and portable. Portable lights are used when fixed lights are not able to reach an area or when additional lighting is necessary. Portable lights generally range from 300 to 1,000 watts. They may be supplied by cords from the power plant or may have self-contained power units. The lights usually have handles for safe carrying and large

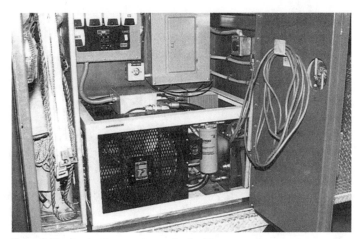

Figure 3-10   An electric generator can be fixed to emergency apparatus.

bases to assure stable placement. Some portable lights are connected to telescoping stands that eliminate the need for personnel either to hold them or to find something to set the lights on.

Fixed lights are mounted on vehicles, and their main function is to provide overall lighting of a large area. Fixed lights are usually mounted so that they can be raised, lowered, or turned to provide the best possible lighting. Often, these lights are mounted on telescoping poles that allow this movement. More elaborate setups include electrically, pneumatically, or hydraulically operated booms with banks of lights (Figure 3-11). Such a bank of lights generally has a capacity of 500 to 1,500 watts per light. The amount of power needed for the lighting should be carefully matched with the amount of power available from the power-generating device carried on the vehicle. Overtaxing the power-generating device will give poor lighting, may damage the power-generating unit or the lights, and will limit the operation of other electrical tools.

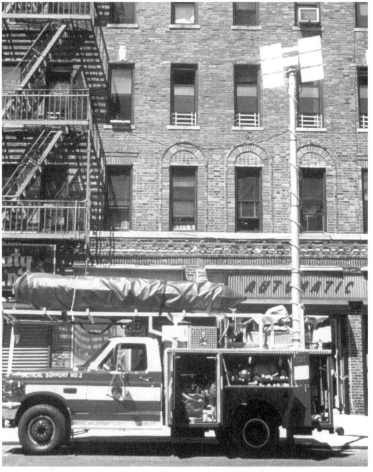

Figure 3-11   Some vehicles are equipped with movable banks of floodlights.

A variety of other electrical distribution equipment may be used in conjunction with power-generating and lighting equipment. Electrical cables or extension cords are necessary to conduct electric power to portable equipment. The most common-size cable is a 12-gauge, 3-wire type. The cord may be stored in coils, on portable cord reels, or on fixed automatic rewind reels. Twist-lock receptacles provide secure, safe connections. Electrical cables must be adequately insulated and waterproofed and must have no exposed wires.

Junction boxes may be used when multiple connections are needed. The junction is supplied by one inlet from the power plant and is fitted with several outlets. Junction boxes are commonly equipped with small lights on top to make them easier to find and plug into in the dark.

Because mutual-aid departments frequently work together and often have different sizes or types of receptacles (for example, one department uses two-prong receptacles, whereas the other uses three-prong devices), adapters should be carried so that equipment can be interchanged. Adapters should also be carried to allow rescuers to plug their equipment into standard electrical outlets.

Rehab Area Marking Equipment

A variety of equipment is available for use in designating and/or cordoning off the rehab area from the rest of the emergency scene. Each jurisdiction tends to have its own method for accomplishing this task, and there is no fixed way that this task must be done. Obviously, agencies that have rehab vehicles will not need to do much more than park a vehicle for responders to determine where the rehab is located. Other agencies may use portable signs or banners to identify the rehab area, or specific points within the rehab area (entry, treatment, etc.).

Once the rehab area has been established and identified, many jurisdictions find it helpful to cordon off the area so that its boundaries are clearly defined. This may be done using traffic cones, vinyl boundary marker tape, rope, or other similar items. Some agencies use a different color of boundary tape for the rehab area than is used elsewhere on the scene. Local SOPs will dictate methods for marking the rehab area as well as what apparatus the marking gear will be carried on. Companies or apparatus that could potentially be assigned to establish the rehab area should carry at least a minimal amount of this equipment to start with.

Misting/Cooling Equipment

Agencies that operate in hot, arid climates often have portable misting or cooling equipment that can be erected in a rehab area to provide some relief for resting firefighters. Two primary types of devices are used for this purpose. The first is a tent-awning or pavilion-type structure that is erected on site. The structural members of this device are piping systems with spray nozzles located around the perimeter of the device. When the system is charged with water, a very fine spray mist is discharged from the nozzles. As this mist hits the hot, arid air, the resulting evaporation can cool the surrounding air by as much as 20°F to 30°F (10°C to 20°C).

The second type of device is a mechanical blower with a water line run into it. A spray nozzle within the unit introduces a water mist into the discharge side of the blower. This device cools both by movement of the air by the fan and by evaporation of the water being blown out of it. Both types of devices work best in climates of low relative humidity. Their cooling effects decrease as the humidity rises.

Both devices obviously require an external water supply. If a device cannot be attached to a municipal water supply or some equivalent, it must be supplied with water by a fire department pumper. Because these devices flow a very low volume of water, often less than 10 gallons per minute (40 liters per minute), a fire department pumper operating off its water tank can supply the device for an extended period of time.

Chairs

Although some responders are perfectly comfortable sitting on the ground while they are resting, many others prefer to sit on chairs or benches during their rehab time. Some agencies carry chairs or benches on their rehab or special service apparatus for use in the rehab area. Remember that the responders using this equipment are often large individuals wearing at least some heavy protective clothing. Chairs carried on apparatus for rehab purposes must therefore be both portable and sturdy. Light-duty, inexpensive folding lawn chairs will probably not last long in rehab. Instead, sturdy folding chairs or stackable, resin-type patio chairs are recommended.

Beverage Serving Equipment

A key function in rehab areas is the dispensing of beverages to the personnel resting there. There are two primary ways this is done. The first is to use individual serving containers, such as bottles of water or cans of sports activity drinks. When individual serving containers are used, it may be necessary to have large coolers of ice available to keep them chilled.

The second method is to use large serving dispensers (Figure 3-12). These are insulated containers inside which water or sports activity drinks and ice are kept. If large serving dispensers are used, disposable cups for personnel will also be required. The advantage of using these containers is cost; their use is usually less expensive than individual containers.

It is generally recommended that cups used for serving beverages have a capacity of at least 16 ounces. Cups of this size allow firefighters to get reasonable-size drinks and then sit down and relax. Smaller cups encourage return visits to the beverage dispenser, which works against the goal of rest and relaxation.

If food service is provided, additional equipment may be required. The amount of equipment will vary with the level of food service the agency wishes to have available at the scene.

It should always be the goal of the Rehab Unit Leader to make sure that the area used for rehab looks at least as good following the operation as it did before the establishment of rehab. With that in mind, trash receptacles should be placed in the rehab area when food or drinks are dispensed. There are many styles of portable or collapsible trash containers that may be carried on response vehicles. An extra supply of trash can liners should also be carried.

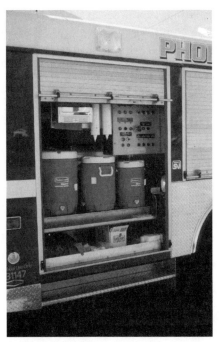

Figure 3-12   Large serving dispensers are extremely useful for rehydrating personnel.

OPERATING A REHAB AREA

Various factors will affect the way a rehab area is actually operated. These include the available staffing, the number of personnel on the scene needing rehab, and local SOPs. Every jurisdiction should develop SOPs for rehab operations that are realistic for the resources available. Jurisdictions that develop grandiose rehab procedures but can only staff the rehab area at an incident with two EMT-Basics (EMT-Bs) are bound to be disappointed in the level of service rehab provides.

Because there are many different jurisdictional approaches to rehab, the material below does not lay out one specific method of staffing and operating a rehab area. Rather, this section focuses on the *functions* that must be performed in a rehab area. How these duties are divided up or delegated is a jurisdiction-specific issue. However, all these functions should be accounted for, in some manner, within each jurisdiction's SOPs for rehab.

Rehab Area Staffing

The Rehab group/sector should be staffed with adequate personnel to provide medical evaluation and treatment and to assure that firefighters receive sufficient fluid replenishment and food. What defines "adequate personnel" varies with the scope of the incident and the number of responders assigned to it.

The most highly trained and qualified EMS personnel on the scene should provide medical evaluation and treatment in the Rehab group/sector. At the minimum, the Medical Evaluation/Treatment Unit should be staffed by EMT-Bs. EMT-Bs assigned to the Rehab group/sector perform several key functions:

- EMT-Bs must assure that the sector provides a safe area in which fire and rescue crews can rest and receive *rehydration*, or replacement of water and electrolytes lost in sweating. During prolonged incidents, food should also be supplied to crews in the rehabilitation area.
- EMT-Bs must identify firefighters and rescue personnel entering the sector who are at risk for heat- and stress-related illness or injury.
- EMT-Bs assigned to rehab should have an automated external defibrillator (AED) readily available in the unlikely, but statistically important, event that a firefighter experiences cardiac arrest.
- EMT-Bs must medically monitor crews and determine whether they:
  Are fit to return to active fire/rescue duty.
  Require additional hydration and rest.
  Require transport to a hospital emergency department for further evaluation and treatment.
- EMT-Bs must assure accountability of firefighters and rescue personnel who enter and exit the sector.
- EMT-Bs must give regular reports/updates to the Safety Officer or the Incident Commander.

In large-scale incidents or in those where a trend toward serious heat- and stress-related illness is detected among firefighters, paramedics and advanced life-support (ALS) units should be requested and assigned to the Rehab group/sector. The role of ALS personnel will be to evaluate and treat those responders in rehab who appear to be in need of a higher level of care than EMT-Bs can provide. This care includes the establishment of IVs for severely dehydrated personnel and advanced care of heat- or stress-related illnesses. Often, non–fire service EMS agencies provide medical evaluation and treatment in the Rehab group/sector. If such agencies are used, it is essential that they have direct radio communication with Command.

In some jurisdictions, personnel assigned to the rehab area will also be responsible for transporting responders needing further care to the hospital. In such cases, enough personnel must be assigned to the Rehab group/sector to assure that it remains fully operational whenever one crew leaves on a transport assignment.

Personnel without emergency medical training can play important parts in rehab operations. They may be used for functions such as providing fluid replenishment and food in the Rehab group/sector. In many jurisdictions, members of the fire department's Ladies' Auxiliary, an Explorer Post, or departmental civilian staff members fill this function. In addition, agencies such as the American Red Cross and Salvation Army, local civic organizations such as the Lion's Club and Rotary Club, or local food retailers may offer additional nutritional support. When such organizations are involved in emergency scene operations, they must follow the directions of Command or the Rehab Unit Leader. This is especially important in order to assure that proper types of fluids—noncarbonated and caffeine-free—are administered.

Entry Point/Initial Assessment

The process of maintaining an effective rehab operation begins by assuring that all personnel enter the Rehab group/sector through a single designated entry point (Figure 3-13). This will allow all responders to be processed in an orderly fashion in which potential problems are not likely to be overlooked. Each person entering the rehab area should be time-logged in by the Rehab Unit Leader or someone else who is delegated that function. Accountability identifiers should also be collected by the log-in person. It is highly recommended that entire crews enter and exit rehab as a group. For example, one exhausted member of Engine 65 should not be sent to rehab alone while the other members continue to perform their duties. The entire company should be assigned to rehab at this point, and its duties should be reassigned to a fresh company.

Upon entering rehab, firefighters should be allowed to remove their SCBAs, hoods, and turnout gear. In hot weather, if turnout pants are not completely removed, they should at least be opened and lowered, allowing heat to dissipate from the lower body. Other responders, such as police tactical team members, should be allowed to remove any bulky clothing or equipment they are wearing. Responders who are working in special protective clothing at hazmat incidents should go

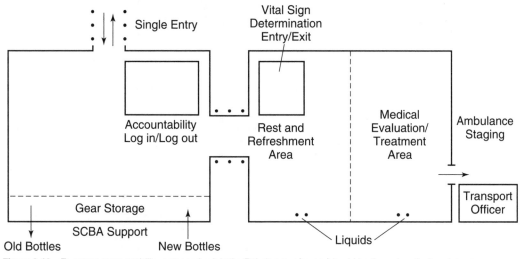

Figure 3-13   To assure accountability, entry and exit in the Rehab group/sector should be through a single point.

through decontamination and remove their special protective clothing at the decontamination area before proceeding to rehab (Figure 3-14).

Once excess gear is removed, each crew member should be evaluated for injuries and for heat- and stress-related illnesses. The first step in evaluation is obtaining entry vital signs, including blood pressure, pulse, and temperature. Rehab staff should rapidly question crew members, being alert to potentially life-threatening complaints such as chest pain or shortness of breath. Remember, the goal of the entry medical evaluation is to identify personnel with potential heat- or stress-related illnesses or injuries, not to keep firefighters from rest and rehydration.

When the entry evaluation is complete, sector staff should assign crew members either to the Rest and Refreshment Unit or to the Medical Evaluation/Treatment Unit. Patients assigned to the Medical Evaluation/Treatment Unit will receive more intensive evaluation and monitoring in addition to rehydration and rest. The findings of the entry medical evaluation determine the area to which crew members are assigned. More information on medical evaluation of responders and the criteria for sending them to the Medical Evaluation/Treatment Unit is contained in Chapter 4. As a general rule, however, any responder with a pulse rate greater than 120 beats per minute, with a body temperature above 100.6°F (38.1°C), or with any injuries should be assigned to the Medical Evaluation/Treatment Unit.

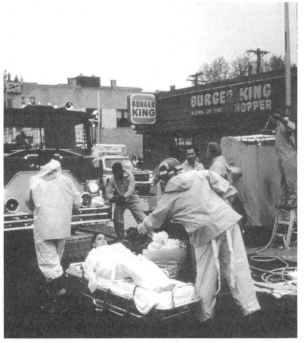

Figure 3-14 During hazmat operations, decontamination should be performed before responders enter the Rehab group/sector.

Rest and Refreshment Unit

Responders who have satisfactory vital signs and no injuries but are simply tired should be directed to the Rest and Refreshment Unit of the Rehab group/sector. There they will be able to rest, drink fluids to replace those lost through sweating, and get food if they are hungry or in need of an energy boost. The person in charge of this area is known as the *Rest Unit Leader.*

In hot weather, if the Rest and Refreshment Unit is in an air-conditioned environment, the responders should be allowed to let their bodies cool down at ambient temperatures for a few minutes before entering the air conditioning. Otherwise, their bodies' cooling systems may shut down in response to the external cooling. In cold weather, there should be no delay in getting responders into a warmer environment.

The amount of time that responders will require in the Rest and Refreshment Unit will vary depending on a variety of conditions, including:

- The responder's level of physical conditioning
- The atmospheric conditions
- The nature of the activities the responder was performing before entering rehab
- The time needed for adequate rehydration and/or eating

It is recommended that departments establish a minimum amount of time for all personnel to spend resting in the rehab area. Local policies will vary depending on normal atmospheric conditions and the number of available responders. A good general rule of thumb, however, is that each person should be allowed at least 20 minutes of rest time on initial entry into rehab. Members who still appear fatigued after that point may be allowed additional rest time. There is no set maximum amount of time that a responder should be allowed to rest. However, any responder who has not recovered sufficiently to return to service within 30 minutes should be sent to the Medical Evaluation/Treatment Unit for a more thorough checkup. There the responder will either receive further treatment or be sent home.

Obviously, the hydration function that occurs in this part of the rehab area is very important to responders' recovery. Personnel who perform heavy work, under stressful conditions, while wearing heavy personal protective clothing are subject to excessive fluid loss. While fluid loss is obvious in hot weather (because of excessive sweating), do not overlook the fact that dehydration also occurs in cold climates. Dehydration is not as evident during cold weather because there may not be as much visible sweat on the responder. That is because cold air tends to have less humidity than warm air, making perspiration more likely to evaporate quickly off the skin. In addition, the many layers of clothing worn by the responder are likely to absorb any perspiration that forms.

Maintaining sufficient levels of water and electrolytes in the body can greatly aid in the prevention of heat- or stress-related illness and injury. Under extreme sweating conditions, responders may need to consume as much as 1 quart (1 liter) of water per hour in order to maintain safe levels in their systems.

Drinks should be easily accessible to responders who are in this area. The drinks may be served in individual serving containers (cans or bottles) or from large service dispensers. If large dispensers are used, there must be an ample supply of large, disposable drinking cups nearby. Responders should be encouraged to drink as much as they feel they need to quench their thirsts and replace the fluids in their bodies. The amount of liquid each person needs will vary.

Serving food at incidents is not as common as serving beverages. In general, it is only necessary to provide food at incidents that extend longer than 3 hours or over a period when a normal meal has been missed. For example, think of an incident that occurs early in the morning, before most or all of the responders have had the opportunity to eat breakfast. It may have been nearly 12 hours since these people had eaten supper the night before. In such a case, it would be necessary to get some food to responders on the scene in a timely manner.

The types of foods served at an emergency scene will vary based on the local customs, the weather conditions (hot food in the winter, cool food during the summer), the time of day, and the capabilities of the food provider. In general, fatty and salty foods should not be served. More specific information on appropriate foods and drinks can be found in Chapter 5.

If the food being served comes in individual packaging—for example, high-energy bars or bananas—no special serving provisions need to be made. If food is prepared on the scene and served in portions—for example, soup, sandwiches, or full meals—the food provider must have appropriate equipment to store the uncooked food, to cook it properly, and to serve it in a sanitary manner. Disposable dishes and utensils should generally be used in these operations because washing dishes is usually impossible at the scene. State or local health department guidelines may apply to these operations

Medical Evaluation/Treatment Unit

Personnel who did not have satisfactory vital signs at entry into rehab, who show obvious signs of illness or injury, or who have not shown signs of appropriate recuperation in the Rest and Refreshment Unit should be immediately sent to the Medical Evaluation/Treatment Unit (hereafter referred to as the *Treatment Unit*). A more thorough examination will be conducted there. More aggressive care procedures, such as the application of cooling devices or the establishment of IVs, can also take place in this area (Figure 3-15). The person in charge of this area is known as the Treatment Unit Leader. If the incident involves multiple casualties not related to the rehab function, it may be desirable to designate this person as the Rehab Treatment Unit Leader. This will avoid confusion with the Treatment Unit Leader who is part of the Medical Branch in the Operations Section.

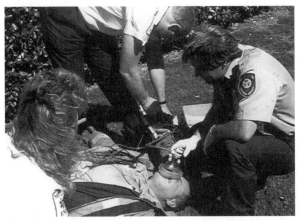

Figure 3-15   More aggressive care can be provided to responders in the Medical Evaluation/Treatment Unit.

The Treatment Unit should be staffed by the highest level of emergency medical care providers on the scene. Ideally, paramedics will be available for staffing. In some jurisdictions, an EMS medical director, fire department physician, or other medical doctor may be available for duties here.

The tasks of the personnel staffing this area include evaluating responders' vital signs, conducting detailed examinations, attempting to recognize potential medical problems as early as possible, and determining the proper disposition for responders. Depending on the circumstances, the proper disposition could include any of the following:

- Returning the responder to duty
- Continuing the rehab treatment that has been started and continuing to monitor the responder
- Initiating advanced medical treatment as well as transport to a hospital

Responders in the Treatment Unit should have access to fluids and food, as their condition allows. In many cases, the symptoms that forced their assignment to the area are easily corrected with fluids and rest. In some instances, however, responders' conditions will not improve without more significant medical intervention. Responders whose signs and/or symptoms indicate potential problems should be treated and transported in accordance with local protocols established by the medical director. Any responders who require advanced life-support procedures, such as intravenous rehydration, must be removed from the action for the duration of the incident.

Appropriate documentation for every responder assigned to the Treatment Unit is essential. The standard forms used on routine EMS calls can be used in the Treatment Unit. The responder's name and agency should be recorded, along with vital signs, pertinent medical complaints, and treatment information. If a responder is eventually transported to a hospital, this paperwork should be given to the transporting crew. If the responder is not transported, the forms should be made part of the incident report.

Personnel who respond favorably to treatment in the Treatment Unit may then be allowed to go to the Rest and Refreshment Unit or to report for reassignment. More detailed information on the medical evaluation and treatment of responders can be found in Chapter 4.

Transportation Unit

Personnel who do not respond favorably to treatment in rehab must be transported to a hospital for further evaluation and more aggressive treatment. This job is the responsibility of the Transportation Unit of the Rehab group/sector. The person in charge of this unit is known as the Transportation Unit Leader. If the incident involves multiple casualties not related to rehab functions, it may be desirable to designate this person as the Rehab Transportation Unit Leader. This will avoid confusion with the Transportation Unit Leader who works in the Medical Branch in the Operations Section.

In some jurisdictions, the transportation function is grouped together with the evaluation/treatment function. While the fit may seem natural, there are excellent reasons why this is not the practice of choice in most jurisdictions. First, it may be disruptive to have personnel who are evaluating/treating numerous responders suddenly have to load one patient up and leave for the hospital. This could affect the care of other responders left in rehab.

The combination of the transportation function with evaluation/treatment also goes against the principles of incident management used in multiple-casualty emergency medical incidents. Agencies accustomed to operating within an incident management system generally find operating the rehab area easier if they follow the same basic principles used with multiple-casualty incidents. Standard IMS procedures at multicasualty incidents call for the Medical Branch to be divided into three distinct Groups or Sectors: Triage, Treatment, and Transportation (Figure 3-16). If you equate the Rehab group/sector with a multiple-casualty situation, parallels to the IMS command structure become evident:

> Entry Point = Triage
> Evaluation/Treatment = Treatment
> Transportation = Transportation

The Transportation Unit Leader is appointed by the Rehab Unit Leader. The Transportation Unit Leader is responsible for determining and arranging all transportation needs for the rehab operation. He or she is also responsible for allo-

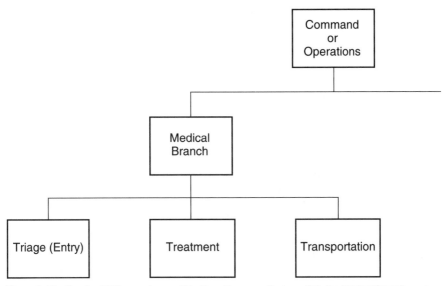

Figure 3-16   Standard IMS procedures call for three Groups or Sectors within the Medical Branch.

cating patients to medical facilities in consultation with the Treatment Unit Leader and personnel at the receiving facilities.

The Transportation Unit Leader is charged with establishing a site from which to manage patient transportation from the rehab area to appropriate medical facilities. The Transportation Unit Leader must "size up" the transportation needs. All requests for transportation resources must then be communicated to the next higher level of supervision. Command will then order the required resources. Once resources are on the scene and assigned to the Transportation Unit, they will report to the Transportation Unit Leader for further direction.

The Transportation Unit Leader must make contact with appropriate medical facilities as soon as possible in order to determine each facility's capacity to receive and treat patients. The leader's initial contact with the facility should include an advisory of the incident situation. This advisory should specify the location of the incident, estimated total number of patients, and estimated number of patients by triage category. Additional information should be forwarded as it is obtained and as time permits. The Transportation Unit Leader should also determine the facility's patient treatment capacity. The appropriate utilization of specialty facilities, such as burn or hyperbaric centers, should be considered when making transport decisions. Medical control hospitals must be advised of the situation, as their standing orders will often be the primary method of treating advanced life-support patients. If it is likely that a large number of responders will require transport, it is essential to communicate this information to the receiving hospital(s) as soon as possible so that the hospital(s) can mobilize the necessary resources and, if necessary, activate an internal disaster plan.

The Treatment Unit advises the Transportation Unit whenever a responder is ready for transport. The Transportation Unit allocates these patients to medical facilities based on the patient's illness or injury, priority, hospital capacity and specialty, and available transportation modes.

Transportation personnel pick patients up from the Treatment Unit when they are ready for transport and deliver them to the selected ambulances or other means of transportation. Patients should not be removed from the Treatment Unit until they are ready for transport. Any documentation begun on the patient in the Treatment Unit should be handed over to transportation personnel during the transfer of patient care. The patient's accountability identifier should be forwarded to the Accountability Officer or to the Incident Commander so that this person is aware that the patient is no longer on the scene. As patients are transported from the scene, hospitals should be advised of estimated arrival times and of basic patient information.

The Transportation Unit Leader must be prepared to assume a proactive stance. Additional resources may be required based on the number of responders to be transported and the complexity of the incident. Additional personnel may be needed for medical communications, transport loading, ground medical transport coordination, record keeping, air medical transport coordination, and ambulance staging. The unit leader must be ready to request these resources ahead of time based on his or her ongoing evaluation of the incident.

The Transportation Unit Leader should be located close to the Treatment Unit Leader since frequent communication and good coordination between these individuals will be necessary. At least two radio channels will be needed for effective transportation operations. Communication between the Transportation Unit and hospitals must be established on a separate radio channel from that used by the Rehab group/sector. This will avoid interference with the tactical channel that is used by the Incident Commander. The Transportation Unit Leader must also maintain communications with the Command post on the tactical channel.

All ambulances must be staged off-site and brought in as needed. Ambulances should go to a single central staging area (preferably the same staging area for all resources responding to the incident) and should be brought to the scene one or two at a time for patient loading. In some situations, a separate ambulance staging area may be required. A Staging Area Manager will be required for each. Provision for transfer to air medical transport—for example, establishment of or conveyance to helicopter landing zones—may also be necessary.

Critical Incident Stress Management

On occasion, the incident that required establishment of a rehab area is one that creates particularly high levels of emotional stress. Such incidents may include:

- Multiple-casualty medical incidents
- Fires with serious injuries or fatalities to civilians or firefighters

- Terrorist incidents
- Long-term hostage situations

Events like these are called *critical incidents.* Such an incident can produce an extreme stress reaction, one so strong that it can interfere with a responder's ability to function, either during the incident or after it. This intense reaction leaves the responder at increased risk of developing long-term emotional and psychological difficulties, including post-traumatic stress syndrome.

To counteract these risks, systems of comprehensive critical incident stress management have been developed. The cornerstone of most of these programs is the process of critical incident stress debriefing (CISD). The elements of CISD carried out while responders are still on the emergency scene are generally done within the Rehab group/sector or Medical Unit.

CISD is a specially organized, open discussion that takes place during and after a serious and emotionally taxing event. Its purpose is to provide a forum in which emergency workers can release their stress. What constitutes a "critical incident" requiring CISD should be determined by the needs of the emergency personnel who were on the scene. For example, in a big city, a motor vehicle crash in which two teenagers are killed may not be perceived as a major incident. In a small rural village, such a crash might emotionally devastate the entire community. Usually the Incident Commander or Medical Unit will initiate the CISD process when the nature of the incident indicates that these services will be required.

Full CISD is a multiple-step process. The step that is usually carried out on the scene, in the Medical Unit, is called a *defusing session.* The defusing session is a shorter form of the debriefing that will come later. The personnel who were involved in the incident and are now in rehab are usually the only participants. The defusing session gives participants a chance to vent their emotions about the incident. The session also can help them get ready for the kind of discussion that will take place in the debriefings that will occur later on. Many jurisdictions prefer to have trained mental health clinicians on the scene to handle this function. Other jurisdictions have emergency response personnel who are trained for conducting this procedure.

At the *debriefing,* a group of specially trained peer counselors and mental health professionals sit down with the emergency workers involved in the incident. All personnel (including those in command of the incident) are encouraged, but should not be forced, to attend. The debriefing should be held within 24 to 72 hours of the incident. At the meeting, an open, confidential discussion of the responders' feelings, fears, and reactions should take place. Table 3-1 shows what the various stages of the CISD aim to accomplish.

CISD is neither an investigation nor an interrogation, nor is it a tactical debriefing. It should be a nonthreatening meeting in which emergency workers can openly express their emotions. The trained professionals who take part can offer concrete suggestions for ways of overcoming the stress related to the incident.

Table 3-1   Phases of a CISD

Phase	Purpose
Introduction	Sets goals for the CISD. Assures confidentiality. Assures that comments won't affect job ratings.
Facts	Sets out details of what occurred at the incident.
Feelings	Encourages participants to explore feelings the incident raised in them.
Symptoms	Encourages participants to note any physical reactions the incident may have caused in them.
Teaching	Allows professionals to help participants sort through feelings. Provides opportunity to reinforce the fact that extreme reactions are normal in such situations.
Reentry	Offers suggestions for coping with stress after the CISD. May include creating an action plan, setting goals, and prescribing activities to reduce stress.
Follow-up	Explores how participants have been coping with the situation some months or weeks later.

CISD is not an absolute cure for the stress related to a major incident. Holding a CISD soon after the incident can, however, accelerate the normal recovery process. It can also reduce or eliminate some stress reactions.

In addition to CISD, a comprehensive critical incident stress management program should include the following components:

- Preincident education about stress and stress reactions
- On-scene peer support of emergency personnel
- One-on-one support as needed
- Disaster support services
- Informal defusing sessions
- Follow-up support services as needed
- Spouse and family support
- Community outreach programs
- Other health and wellness programs based on local needs and resources
- Religious counseling/services (chaplain)

Reassignment Unit

Personnel who are released from the Rehab group/sector will find themselves subject to one of three dispositions:

1. They will be transported to a hospital for further evaluation and treatment.
2. They will be reassigned to another function on the emergency scene.
3. They will be returned to regular service and sent back to the station.

Obviously, personnel who are transported to a hospital will not make it to the Reassignment Unit. The Reassignment Unit deals primarily with responders who are ready to return to incident operations or who may be released to return to service. The person in charge of the Reassignment Unit is known as the Reassignment Unit Leader. On smaller incidents, the Rehab Unit Leader may perform this function personally. In larger, more complex operations, the Rehab Unit Leader assigns someone to handle this task. In either case, the person handling this function must be capable of making a sound medical judgment about the readiness of each responder to return to incident activities.

Personnel who are being considered for reassignment should appear rested and must have satisfactory vital signs. (More information on appropriate vital signs and responder conditions may be found in Chapter 4.) The Reassignment Unit Leader should confirm the responders' readiness with the Rest Unit Leader and/or the Treatment Unit Leader. Keep in mind that the responders should have entered rehab as a crew. They should not be returned to service unless the entire crew is ready for service.

However, on some occasions, an entire crew may not be ready to return to service at the same time. For example, perhaps three of four crew members are fit and ready for service, but the fourth member required transport to a hospital. In this case, the Reassignment Unit Leader has several options for the remaining crew members:

- If the fourth member was severely injured or ill, it may be better to remove the rest of the members of the crew from service and allow them to direct their attention to the well-being of their colleague.
- The crew could be reassigned to a function that can be handled by a three-person crew. If the missing crew member was the leader or company officer, one of the remaining members should be designated as the new leader.
- The remaining crew members could be assigned to be part of another crew under a different leader.

When a crew is ready for service, the Reassignment Unit Leader should notify the Incident Commander, Operations Section Chief, or Staging Officer that the crew is available. The size of the incident and the complexity of the IMS that is in place will determine which of these three is to be notified. There are generally four options for a full crew that is ready for service:

1. If the crew is no longer needed at the incident, the members are returned to regular service. They should collect any equipment they have used on the emergency scene, restore their apparatus to a state of readiness, and return to quarters.
2. If there is an immediate need for the crew on the emergency scene, the crew should be given a new assignment. Included in its assignment should be an explanation of which command officer it will be reporting to, the radio channel it will be operating on, and the accountability officer that it should report to for that part of the operation. At this time, the Reassignment Unit Leader should return the accountability identifiers to the crew members, note their release on the log sheet, and send them to their destination.
3. *For incidents where a separate staging area has been established:* If a crew is not immediately needed to perform another function on the scene but its participation is

anticipated at a later time, it should be released from the Rehab group/sector and advised to report to Staging. At this point, the Reassignment Unit Leader should return the accountability identifiers to the crew members, note their release on the log sheet, and send them to Staging.

4. *For incidents where no separate staging area has been established:* If the crew is not immediately needed to perform another function on the scene but it may be needed later, it should remain in the Rest and Refreshment Unit or Reassignment Unit of the Rehab group/sector until it is given another assignment. When it receives that assignment, the Reassignment Unit Leader should return the accountability identifiers to the crew members, note their release on the log sheet, and send them to their destination.

Demobilizing Rehab Group/Sector Operations

The Rehab Unit Leader must maintain constant communication with the Incident Commander to determine when it will be possible to begin scaling down rehab operations. Keep in mind that even though an incident such as a fire may be brought under control, often the most physically demanding work, such as overhaul, still remains. There will generally be a need for some form of rehab to continue until all responders have left the scene.

As responders begin to leave the incident scene, the number of personnel assigned to each function within the Rehab group/sector may be reduced correspondingly. However, adequate staffing must be maintained to assure that all rehab services are still available to those responders who remain on the scene.

As each company or apparatus that was assigned to the Rehab group/sector returns to service, its member should make sure that all equipment they brought with them is properly stowed. An inventory of expendable supplies that were used at the incident should be taken and every effort made to restock as soon as possible. The next incident requiring rehab may take place in 5 months or 5 minutes, so readiness is essential.

For both public relations and safety considerations, the location where rehab operated should be restored to a condition equal to or better than what it was before operations began. All trash should be collected and disposed of properly. Any spent medical supplies should also be collected and disposed of following local protocols. Any areas where food was dispensed should be cleaned so that animals or insects do not gather there.

4

MEDICAL ASPECTS OF REHAB OPERATIONS

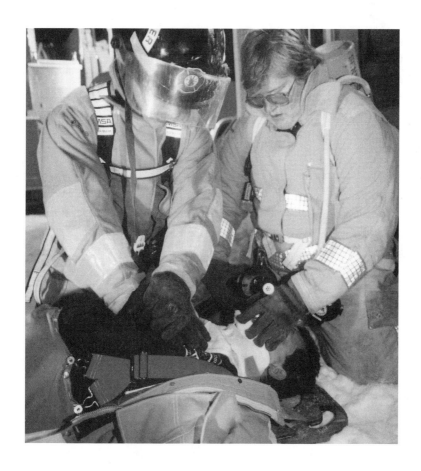

Firefighters die of stress- and heat-related illnesses far more often than they do of burns or injuries suffered in structural collapses. Although fire fighting is an inherently hazardous, physically demanding occupation, appropriate emergency scene rehabilitation that incorporates appropriate medical monitoring and interventions can reduce the risks of stress- and heat-related illnesses and deaths associated with fire fighting and other emergency scene operations.

PRINCIPLES GUIDING REHAB OPERATIONS

Several key principles should guide rehab medical operations at emergency scenes. They include the following:

- Keep all firefighters well hydrated and rested to minimize their risks of developing heat- and stress-related illnesses.
- Provide ongoing medical monitoring in order to identify as early as possible those rescue workers who show any signs of the development of stress- or heat-related illnesses.
- During initial or ongoing medical monitoring, rapidly identify any potentially serious medical conditions and initiate treatment of them.
- Treat any traumatic injuries detected.
- After appropriate rehabilitation and medical monitoring have been provided, assure each firefighter is appropriately triaged with one of the following dispositions:
  1. The firefighter is adequately rehabbed and medically "sound" for return to duty.
  2. The firefighter has ongoing signs of illness or an injury that mandate that he or she remain in Rehab and/or be removed from duty.
  3. The firefighter requires transportation to an appropriate medical facility for further evaluation and treatment of illness or injury.

In order for the medical personnel assigned to rehab to carry out their tasks efficiently, rehab operations must be seamlessly integrated into the Incident Command System. A key element of the ICS structure is the willingness of Command to support the medical decisions made by emergency medical personnel who are evaluating and treating firefighters. Medical personnel must have the authority to determine which firefighters are fit to return to emergency operations and which personnel must remain in rehab or even be transported for further medical evaluation (Figure 4-1). Individual egos and "macho"-based overruling of medical personnel will ultimately result in the same dire consequences as any other "freelancing" within the ICS structure.

It is important to remember that the medical monitoring and emergency medical care provided in the Rehab sector must be distinguished from general EMS care provided at the incident scene. Civilian casualties or overt medical or trauma emergencies involving firefighters that occur on the fireground or on the rescue scene should be treated and transported from the scene by EMS units assigned to the Medical Sector to cover such occurrences. For example, firefighters injured in a wall

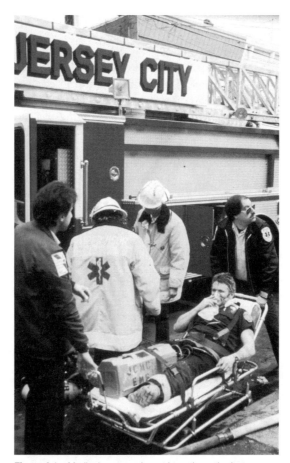

Figure 4-1 Medical personnel must have the authority to decide if responders are medically fit to return to scene operations, or need transport for additional medical evaluation or care.

collapse should be treated and transported from the scene by Medical Sector personnel rather than being sent to Rehab to be cared for by medical personnel assigned to that area. Often, the Medical and Rehab sectors will share a common ambulance staging area to facilitate the smooth transport of patients from the scene. However, the injuries and medical emergencies treated in the Rehab sector are usually only the ones detected upon firefighters' entry into the area or those that subsequently develop while firefighters are in Rehab.

Although this chapter focuses primarily on medical evaluation and treatment performed by medical personnel in the rehab area, keep in mind that *all* firefighters have an obligation to act as "medical monitors" while on the fireground or emergency scene, even if they are not actually assigned to work in the Rehab sector. As a firefighter, you must always be alert to your own physical and mental limitations when on duty. You should also look out for the physical and emotional well-being of your fellow firefighters. If you identify signs of illness or detect an injury in a fellow firefighter, you should advise your company officer or Command of the situation so that your company can be moved into Rehab for further evaluation and/or treatment. Similarly, if you suffer an injury or begin to feel ill, you should advise your fellow firefighters and officer of the situation. A macho firefighter who puts his or her ego ahead of a willingness to admit to illness or injury not only puts himself or herself at risk but also endangers the well-being of fellow firefighters. This is especially true when a situation arises that requires immediate physical and mental response that the firefighter may not be capable of due to illness or injury. Remember that an exhausted firefighter risks not only his or her own life but the lives of others as well. If you feel you are at your physical or psychological limits or see others who appear to be at theirs, your crew must report to the Rehab group/sector for rest and evaluation.

INJURIES AND ILLNESSES AT EMERGENCY INCIDENT SCENES

It is important to understand what types of injuries and illnesses you are likely to encounter in the Rehab area. Table 4-1 illustrates several key points about the emergency medical aspects of the Rehab sector. These points can be summarized as follows:

1. Injuries, including burns, cuts, bruises, strains, sprains, and fractures, are the most common conditions encountered in rehab.
2. Smoke- and gas-related inhalation injuries account for about 1 out of 10 duty-related injuries (despite mandated use of SCBA).
3. Thermal stress is a common mechanism of illness.
4. Strokes and heart attacks generally account for less than 1 percent of illnesses, but represent 50 percent of on-duty deaths among firefighters.

Table 4-1   Firefighter Injuries by Nature of Injury and Type of Duty (1996)

Nature of Injury	Fireground		Nonfire Emergency	
	Number	Percent	Number	Percent
Burns (fire or chemical)	4,360	9.5	140	1.1
Smoke or gas inhalation	4,660	10.2	305	2.4
Other respiratory distress	740	1.6	210	1.6
Eye irritation	2,735	6.0	390	3.1
Wound (cut, bleeding, bruise)	8,775	19.2	2,055	16.3
Dislocation, fracture	1,090	2.4	260	2.0
Heart attack or stroke	300	0.7	45	0.4
Strain, sprain, muscular pain	17,455	38.2	7,020	55.6
Thermal stress (frostbite, heat exhaustion)	2,270	5.9	185	1.5
Other	2,890	6.3	2,020	16.0
Total	45,725		12,630	

Traumatic Injuries Encountered in Rehab

Traumatic injuries are the most common conditions encountered by medical personnel in the rehab sector. The majority of these injuries—cuts, muscular strains, and minor burns—are generally not immediately life-threatening and can readily be treated in accordance with basic life support measures.

Key aspects of management of the injuries encountered in the Rehab sector include the following:

- Wounds that are grossly contaminated with debris such as soot or other charred particles should be irrigated with copious amounts of water or saline solution in the Rehab sector to remove as much contaminated material from the wound as possible before bandaging. Doing this will reduce the risk of subsequent wound infections.
- Burns should be treated as directed by local EMS system protocols. Generally, burns involving less than 10 percent of body surface area (BSA) are treated with moist sterile dressings. Burns involving more than 10 percent BSA are dressed with dry sterile dressings, once it has been assured that any residual burning of tissue has been extinguished.
- Eye injuries are common. The most common eye emergencies are caused by debris striking the eyes. This will often produce very painful corneal injuries, usually in the form of abrasions. Since loss or serious impairment of vision can be a career-ending, life-altering event, meticulous on-scene eye care is essential. Follow these basic care steps, or your local protocols, with cases of eye injury:

  Irrigate any visible particles from the eye with sterile saline or clean water. Patch the affected eye closed to reduce the risk of further injury caused by the eye's movement. Some local protocols recommend patching both eyes. If both eyes are patched, the patient must be constantly reassured and never left alone. Some advanced life support EMS systems allow the use of topical eye anesthetics to reduce pain and the insertion of eye irrigation devices (such as a Morgan lens) during transport to the hospital.

  If there is chemical exposure to the eye, irrigate both on-scene and while en route to the hospital. Eyes with serious chemical exposure should not be patched, as doing this may hold residual chemicals more closely to the surface of the eye.

  Any lacerations or potential ruptures of the globe of the eye should be immediately covered with a rigid eye shield to reduce the risk of further trauma to the eye.

When determining whether a firefighter with a "minor" injury should be allowed to return to active on-scene duty, always consider the following criteria:

- Any firefighter with an injury that may be worsened by a return to duty should not be allowed to return. For example, a firefighter with wounds that might become further contaminated, thereby increasing the risk of subsequent infection, should not be allowed back on duty.
- Any firefighter with an injury that might in any way impair the performance of his or her duty should not be allowed to return to duty. Example: A firefighter with a minor sprained ankle who would not be able to climb a ladder efficiently should not be reassigned to duty.

Medical Emergencies Encountered in Rehab

Throughout this text, we have mentioned stress- and heat-related emergencies and illnesses. This section discusses specific medical conditions and medical emergencies included in that generic grouping.

Stress-Related Illness

The term *stress* is widely used. From a medical perspective, stress has been traditionally divided into two broad categories, *psychological* stress and *physical* or *physiological* stress.

Psychological Stress   Although this distinction would seem to split stress into either psychological or physiological, there is a growing body of medical evidence that the two are actually closely related. A common expression of this relationship is the concept of "mind over body." It is clear that the sounder a person's mind and the less psychological stress imposed on him or her, the healthier that person is, both physically and mentally. The converse is also true. Consider, for example, the effects of mental stress imposed on a person by the loss of a spouse. Statistics show that 50 percent of people who lose a spouse will have a life-threatening illness within 6 months of the spouse's death.

Hopefully, firefighters will not encounter psychological stressors of the magnitude of a spouse's death while on duty. Nonetheless, there is little doubt that fire fighting is, by its nature, a psychologically stressful occupation. These stressors take many forms—for example, the constant worry about one's personal safety, the recurrent stress of caring for ill and injured patients during EMS responses, or the stress experienced by line officers who are responsible for many other firefighters in dangerous situations (Figure 4-2).

The links between psychological stress and physical well-being appear to occur on various levels within the human body. These include:

- Suppression of the body's immune system and the reduction of its ability to fight off infections
- An alteration in the perception of the severity of pain
- A decrease in the body's ability to mobilize the "fight or flight" response of the sympathetic nervous system
- Alterations in appetite that may further impair physical well-being by establishing a poor baseline nutritional status

Because of the impact that mental stress may have, it is important that rehab operations be able to provide an appropriate level of psychological—as well as physical—rehabilitation and care. Steps to attenuate on-scene stress may include:

- Isolation of the rehabilitation area from visual stressors such as body recovery operations or field morgues

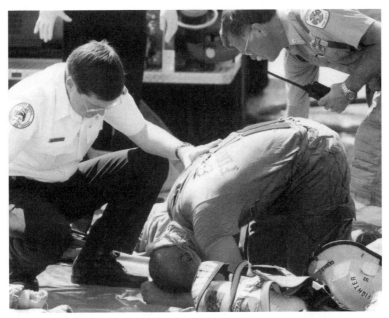

Figure 4-2   Any firefighter can be overwhelmed by the effects of stress at emergency operations.

- Staffing of the rehab area with some personnel who can provide on-scene "diffusing" and early critical incident stress debriefing for psychologically stressed personnel
- Appropriate use of CISD during prolonged operations or at the conclusion of limited, but stressful, operations

During the initial assessment and ongoing monitoring of firefighters in the rehab area, medical personnel should be alert for signs of acute stress reactions. Signs of acute stress include the following:

- Inappropriate expressions of anger
- Aggressive behavior toward other personnel
- Uncontrolled crying or screaming
- Overt signs of depression such as a blunted response to others or the environment

A firefighter demonstrating *any* of these signs of acute stress reaction should not be allowed to return to duty.

Physiological Stress   Physical activity places stresses on the human body. It should then be clear that the bodies of firefighters experience extremely high levels of stress during fire fighting and other rescue operations. These levels of physiological stress are likely to account for many of the firefighter deaths attributed to heart attacks and stroke.

Statistics show that half of all fireground-related deaths are the result of sudden death, acute myocardial infarctions (heart attacks), strokes, and other cardiopulmonary emergencies. For this reason, a discussion of cardiovascular diseases and their associated medical emergencies is warranted here. An understanding of how physiological stresses like those endured by firefighters, can exacerbate such conditions, sometimes with fatal consequences is an important part of that discussion.

Cardiopulmonary Emergencies   The cardiopulmonary system is made up of the heart, lungs, and related structures. Proper functioning of this system depends on adequate functioning of the lungs to assure both the delivery of oxygen to the body and the removal of accumulated carbon dioxide (CO_2) from the bloodstream. In addition, the heart must pump efficiently to assure adequate perfusion of all organ systems in the body. Adequate perfusion of the body's organs with oxygen and adequate removal of carbon dioxide and other waste products will permit the body to function both under normal conditions and during periods of high physiological stress. If the adequacy of breathing or organ perfusion is compromised by acute illness, injury, or a chronic disease such as atherosclerotic heart disease, however, the person's life will be in danger.

In North America, coronary artery disease remains a leading killer of both men and women. In coronary artery disease, the arteries that supply perfusion to the heart muscle become progressively narrowed over time. Deposits of abnormal materials, including cholesterol and other debris, result in a narrowing that eventually reduces the flow of blood to the heart muscle. Reduced blood flow to the heart can result in cardiac emergencies such as *angina pectoris* (severe chest pain), *acute myocardial infarction* (heart attack), and in some cases sudden death from *dysrhythmias,* or irregular electrical activity within the heart's electrical conduction system.

Firefighters with preexisting coronary artery disease are at particular risk for developing cardiac emergencies during periods of physiological stress on the fireground or rescue scene. The reason this is so is that during periods of physical stress, the heart beats faster to provide more blood flow to the body's organs. When the heart beats faster, it requires a greater blood flow through the coronary arteries to supply the increased oxygen demands of the heart adequately. If the coronary arteries have been narrowed by preexisting disease, the heart muscle's demand for blood flow may exceed the ability of the diseased blood vessels to supply it. This lack of blood flow and the accompanying lack of adequate oxygen to permit proper heart muscle function is called *ischemia.* Cardiac ischemia often results in chest pain (angina pectoris) and/or a sensation of shortness of breath. In addition, the heart's electrical system is more likely to function improperly when the heart is ischemic. This can result in cardiac dysrhythmias. In some cases, blood flow through the coronary arteries may become completely blocked, which creates not only ischemia but also *infarction,* or death of cardiac tissue. In this situation, a heart attack or acute myocardial infarction (AMI) may occur. A firefighter who experiences an AMI is at extreme risk for sudden lethal dysrhythmias and sudden death. Therefore, personnel staffing the Rehab group/sector should be aware of the signs and symptoms of cardiac emergencies. These include the following:

- Chest pain or tightness
- Shortness of breath
- Unusually rapid, slow, or irregular pulse or the sensation of palpitations

Any firefighter in whom signs or symptoms of a cardiac emergency are detected upon entry into Rehab should be moved to the Medical Evaluation/Treatment Unit and placed under the care of ALS personnel. The cornerstones of the management of cardiac emergencies include the administration of high-concentration oxygen, cardiac monitoring with an EKG monitor, the ability to provide rapid defibrillation if ventricular fibrillation develops, and the availability of advanced life support medications. Rapid transportation to the nearest appropriate medical facility is mandatory for all cardiac emergency patients.

Stroke Emergencies   Along with heart attacks, strokes are major killers of on-duty firefighters. Strokes, or cerebrovascular accidents (CVAs), most commonly result from the blockage of a cerebral artery in the brain. A small clot or blockage that has traveled through the bloodstream lodges in an artery supplying blood to a certain part of the brain, much like the conditions leading to a heart attack. The flow of blood to the parts of the brain normally supplied by that artery will then be quickly affected. The signs and symptoms that the stroke patient presents will depend on the area of the brain to which blood flow has been disturbed. A common sign of stroke is the presence of drooping on one side of the face and weakness of the arm and/or leg on the opposite side of the body from the facial droop. A person with an acute stroke will often have difficulty speaking due either to slurred speech or to an inability to get the right words out, despite the person's wish to do so.

Any firefighter with signs or symptoms consistent with stroke upon entry into Rehab should be moved immediately to the Medical Evaluation/Treatment Unit of Rehab, and plans for rapid transportation to the hospital should be made. All stroke patients should receive supplemental oxygen and care by ALS personnel. Assuring an open airway and providing adequate ventilations for patients with inadequate breathing are essential to optimizing the chances for the best possible recovery for stroke patients.

A recent major advance in stroke therapy has been the use of *thrombolytics* (like those used in cases of acute heart attack) designed to reopen blocked arteries in the brain. Currently, stroke patients who are within 3 hours of the onset of their symptoms may qualify for this specialized treatment. It is, therefore, essential that medical personnel in Rehab recognize the signs of stroke and be ready to provide rapid transport to a hospital emergency department. There the patient will undergo a rapid screening process that includes an emergency CT scan of the brain prior to the final decision on use of the "clot-busting" drugs.

Heat-Related Emergencies

Heat-related emergencies are among the most common medical conditions encountered in the Rehab group/sector. As has already been noted, the risks of developing one of these conditions are greatly enhanced when personnel are operating in hot and humid environments.

Mechanisms of Heat Loss   Heat loss through *convection* occurs when cooler air moves across the body and the body's heat is transferred to the moving air. The moving air sweeps away the thin layer of warmed air surrounding the body and permits the body to lose heat.

Heat loss through *evaporation* occurs when warmed body moisture is lost to the environment. Evaporative heat loss occurs with normal breathing as warm, moist air is exhaled. Most evaporative heat loss, however, occurs during the process of perspiration. As the body generates heat, it releases a warmed fluid—sweat. The sweat then evaporates into the air, cooling the body surface. The more the body sweats, the more heat is lost.

There are limits to the effectiveness of these heat-loss mechanisms. Convection works as cooler air moves heat away from the body. As the environmental temperature approaches the body's temperature, convectional cooling becomes less effective. For sweat to evaporate and cool the body, the air surrounding the skin has to be relatively low in humidity. As humidity increases, heat loss through evaporation decreases.

Heat-related emergencies are common in fire fighting for several reasons. First, fires emit heat. In structural or wildland fires, heavy fire loads may produce extreme heat. Also, the intense physical activity associated with fire fighting causes firefighters' bodies to generate increased heat. Finally, the protective clothing worn by firefighters, although essential for safety, impairs heat loss through evaporation and convection (Figure 4-3). The combination of high temperatures radiated by fires, increased heat produced by firefighters' bodies, and diminished heat loss because of protective gear places crews fighting fires at serious risk for heat-related emergencies.

The three most important heat-related emergencies that the EMTs will encounter in the Rehab group/sector are heat cramps, heat exhaustion, and heat stroke. Of these conditions, heat stroke is the most serious. Failure to recognize the signs and symptoms of heat stroke and to begin aggressive care may result in the firefighter's death.

Heat Cramps   Heat cramps usually develop during strenuous activity in a hot environment. Excessive sweating results in loss of electrolytes (especially sodium), which contributes to muscle cramping. Heat cramps are usually not a serious problem. They respond well to rest in a cool environment and replacement of fluids by mouth. If a person with heat cramps is untreated and continues to lose fluid because of sweating, heat exhaustion may develop.

Heat Exhaustion   Heat exhaustion occurs when excessive sweat loss and inadequate oral hydration cause depletion of the body's fluid volume. The end result is hypoperfusion of the body's organs. The signs and symptoms of heat exhaustion may vary with the amount of fluid lost. Early signs may include fatigue, light-headedness,

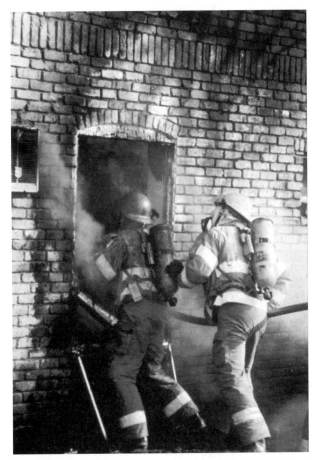

Figure 4-3 Protective clothing worn by firefighters can increase the risk of heat-related emergencies.

nausea, vomiting, and headache. The firefighter's skin is usually pale and moist to the touch, with a cool or normal temperature. If the condition is unrecognized and untreated, a firefighter with heat exhaustion may develop more classic signs of shock or hypoperfusion. These signs include increased heart rate, increased respiratory rate, and—eventually—reduced blood pressure.

Firefighters who engage in structural and wildland fire suppression without adequate rehabilitation often suffer from heat exhaustion. The condition is also common in hazardous materials operations in which firefighters wear encapsulating suits.

Heat Stroke   Heat stroke occurs when the body can no longer regulate its own temperature in hot conditions. Unlike emergency personnel with heat exhaustion whose temperatures are normal or only slightly elevated, those with heat stroke have very high temperatures [up to 106° or 107°F (41° to 41.7°C)]. Because of the high temperature, the skin is likely to feel hot and either dry or moist. The firefighter with heat stroke will have an altered mental status. That mental status may range from mild confusion to complete unresponsiveness.

Any emergency personnel found in a hot environment with altered mental status and skin that is hot and dry or moist to touch should be presumed to have a life-threatening heat-related emergency. Such a patient should be aggressively cooled (see below).

Emergency Care of Heat-Related Emergencies

Firefighters found at an emergency scene who exhibit any of the following symptoms should be treated for a heat-related emergency:

- Muscle cramps
- Weakness or exhaustion
- Dizziness or faintness
- Chest pain
- Shortness of breath
- Rapid heartbeat
- Skin that is
  Normal-to-cool in temperature, pale, moist
  or
  Hot in temperature, dry or moist (a life-threatening sign)
- Headache
- Seizures
- Altered mental status ranging from mild confusion to unresponsiveness (a life-threatening sign)

All firefighters with suspected heat-related emergencies should receive the following treatment:

1. Remove the firefighter from the hot environment; remove any protective clothing including hoods, turnout coats, and bunker pants, and place the person in a cool environment. The air-conditioned patient compartment of an ambulance is ideal.
2. Administer high-flow oxygen.

In cases of apparent heat exhaustion, where the skin is normal-to-cool in temperature, moist to the touch, and pale in color, treat as follows:

1. Remove the firefighter's protective clothing, including headgear, to allow cooling.
2. Cool the firefighter by fanning. Use an electric-powered fan to assist in cooling. Some departments use precooled terry cloth hoods or towels to assist in cooling.
3. Place the firefighter in a supine position with legs elevated.
4. If the firefighter is responsive and not nauseated, have him or her drink water or other fluids as specified by local protocol.

5. If the firefighter is nauseated or vomiting, give nothing by mouth. If ALS personnel are on-scene, initiate an IV of normal saline solution and begin aggressive rehydration. About 1 to 2 liters of IV fluid should be administered. Obtain medical direction for the volume to be infused if required to do so by local protocol.

6. If the firefighter is not responsive, initiate IV fluids and cardiac monitoring and transport the firefighter to the hospital, monitoring and maintaining the airway during transport.

7. Perform the ongoing assessment en route to the hospital.

Any firefighter who presents to the rehab sector with signs or symptoms of heat exhaustion may not return to active duty at the incident. Whether the firefighter will require transport to a medical facility will depend upon local protocols and SOPs, the remoteness of the scene, and the patient's response to rehydration—either oral or by IV—with solutions containing electrolytes.

In cases of apparent heat stroke, where the firefighter's skin is hot and dry or moist to the touch, treat the patient as follows (Figure 4-4):

1. Remove the firefighter's protective clothing, including headgear, to allow cooling.
2. Apply cold packs to the firefighter's neck, groin, and armpits.
3. Keep the skin wet by applying cool water with sponges or wet towels or by wrapping the person in sheets soaked in cool water.
4. Fan aggressively.
5. Use the maximum setting on the air conditioner in the patient compartment of the ambulance.

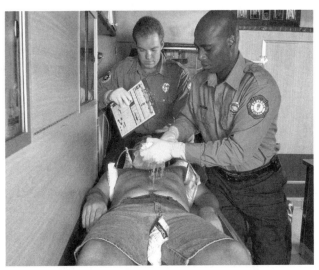

Figure 4-4   With heat stroke, cool aggressively by applying cool packs to the firefighter's neck, armpits, and groin and by applying cool water with sponges or towels. At the same time, fan the firefighter aggressively.

6. Give the firefighter nothing by mouth. Initiate IV fluid administration of normal saline if ALS personnel are present.
7. Transport immediately.
8. Perform an ongoing assessment en route to the hospital.

If not appropriately managed, heat stroke will likely result in the firefighter's death. Early recognition of the condition and rapid cooling are essential to survival in cases of heat stroke.
Remember, the firefighter's survival and recovery from any heat-related emergency hinges on your recognizing the emergency, quickly removing the firefighter from the hot environment, and initiating the proper treatment in the out-of-hospital setting.

Cold-Weather Emergencies

Cold temperatures can result in a variety of illnesses and injuries. The type of cold emergency sustained by a firefighter will depend on a variety of factors, including any preexisting medical conditions or medications as well the type and length of cold exposure. Cold-related emergencies are usually divided into two major types: generalized cold emergencies, which include generalized hypothermia, and localized cold injuries, which include frostbite. Both generalized hypothermia and localized cold injuries may be encountered in the Rehab sector during prolonged cold-weather operations.

Generalized Hypothermia Generalized hypothermia is usually defined as the lowering of body temperature below 95°F (35°C). Generalized hypothermia may be mild or severe. The signs and symptoms encountered vary with the severity of the hypothermia. Generalized hypothermia can occur in a variety of settings. The belief that hypothermia can only occur in extreme winter conditions is untrue. For example, a firefighter involved in springtime flood-relief operations who gets his or her gear wet and is recurrently exposed to 40°F water and ambient air with a temperature of 50°F can easily develop generalized hypothermia.
Signs and symptoms of generalized hypothermia may be detected during entry screening of firefighters into the Rehab sector. Medical personnel assigned to Rehab during operations in which environmental conditions pose a risk of generalized hypothermia to firefighters must be alert to the signs and symptoms of hypothermia including:

- Low or absent blood pressure.
- Slowly responding pupils.
- Presence or absence of shivering.
- Muscle rigidity or a stiff posture.
- Altered mental status. Note that as hypothermia progresses, a patient's mental status declines. Early in hypothermia, patients may exhibit subtle mood changes. Poor coordination, problems with memory, speech difficulties, dizziness, and reduced or lost sensation may also be present in hypothermia. Poor judgment may actually

cause the patient to remove his clothing. Eventually, as hypothermia becomes severe, the patient may become difficult to arouse or completely unresponsive.
- Breathing may be abnormally rapid early on but then becomes abnormally slow as body temperature drops.
- The pulse is often rapid early in hypothermia but becomes abnormally slow as body temperature falls. The pulse rate may be less than 30 beats per minute in advanced hypothermia. The pulse may even be difficult to palpate due to decreased circulation to the extremities. Using the skin to assess circulation is very unreliable in generalized hypothermia, as it is often pale or blue-gray in color due to the direct effects of the cold on the skin.

It is likely that firefighters with generalized hypothermia will meet criteria for immediate transport from Rehab either because of a poor general impression, altered mental status, or inadequate breathing and circulation.

Determining the precise temperature of the firefighter in the field may be difficult. Some EMS agencies carry traditional mercury, electronic, or tympanic thermometers. Although these devices are useful in the assessment of heat-related emergencies, they may be unreliable or impractical during the assessment of the hypothermic firefighter. Rather than using a thermometer, medical personnel should place the backs of their hands between the firefighter's clothing and abdomen during generalized hypothermia assessment. If the abdomen feels cold, then it should be presumed that the patient is hypothermic.

Emergency Medical Care of Generalized Hypothermia   It is neither practical nor safe to attempt complete rewarming of the firefighter in the field. The goals of prehospital care are to remove the patient from the environment, protect the patient from further heat loss, assure an open airway, and support the patient's breathing and circulation. In all aspects of emergency care, handle the hypothermic firefighter extremely gently. Gentle handling is essential because the heart can become irritable in hypothermia. Rough handling can result in cardiac arrest, often from dysrythmias such as ventricular fibrillation.

The exact care a hypothermic firefighter should receive is based upon the his or her mental status—upon whether the firefighter is alert and responding appropriately or whether the firefighter is unresponsive or not responding appropriately. All firefighters suspected of having generalized hypothermia should be treated as follows:

1. Remove the firefighter from the cold environment.
2. Handle the firefighter as gently as possible.
3. Prevent further heat loss by:
   - Removing any cold, wet, or restrictive turnout gear or clothing.
   - Applying warm blankets.
   - Turning the heat up high in the ambulance patient compartment.
4. Maintain an open airway. Suction as needed.

5. Support breathing and circulation. Because respirations and pulse may be very slow, assess the patient for the presence of pulse and breathing for 30 to 45 seconds before starting CPR.
6. Administer high-flow oxygen if not already applied in initial assessment. The oxygen should be warmed and humidified if possible.
7. Do not allow the firefighter to try to walk or exert himself or herself.
8. Do not allow the firefighter to eat or drink stimulants.
9. Do not massage the extremities.

Removing wet or cold clothing, applying warm blankets, and turning the heat in the patient compartment up high are activities that are considered *passive rewarming*. In other words, they allow the firefighter's own body to gradually rewarm itself in a warm environment. All hypothermic firefighters should receive passive rewarming

Active rewarming is the application of external heat to assist the body in rewarming. Active rewarming raises the body temperature more quickly than passive rewarming, but it is a less safe procedure. Although local protocols may vary, passive rewarming should be used only when the hypothermic firefighter is alert and responding appropriately. The active rewarming technique raises the body temperature by warming the blood in major arteries as they pass close to the body's surface in the neck, groin, and axillary regions.

The procedure for active rewarming is as follows:

1. Follow all steps for the general management of the hypothermic firefighter as outlined above.
2. Assure that the firefighter is alert and responding appropriately.
3. Apply heat packs or warm water bottles to the firefighter's groin, axillary, and cervical regions.
4. ALS providers may be allowed by local protocol to administer warmed IV fluid as part of active rewarming.

Prevention of Generalized Hypothermia   Firefighters will always conduct emergency operations in adverse weather conditions. The risk of firefighters developing generalized hypothermia can be greatly reduced by intergrating certain routine procedures in cold-weather operations. These steps should include:

- Rotation of firefighters out of cold and cool environments into warmed cabs of apparatus, into patient compartments of ambulances, or even into running and warm commercial or school buses. On some scenes, there may be an appropriate structure nearby that can house the rehab sector.
- Provision of dry sets of turnout gear for soaked firefighters involved in prolonged operations.

Local Cold Injuries   Firefighters will often suffer the effects of exposure to the cold without developing generalized hypothermia. Local cold injuries are most frequently the result of inadequately protected body parts. The parts of the body farthest from its core are at the greatest risk of injury. The ears, nose, and other parts of the face are most commonly injured. Local cold injuries of the extremities, especially the toes, are also common.

Many of the same predisposing factors that place firefighters at risk for generalized hypothermia also increase the risk of local cold injuries. Any condition, such as diabetes or exhaustion, that decreases a person's ability to sense the cold will increase the risk of local cold injury. In addition, firefighters and other rescue personnel who are significantly dehydrated may also be at increased risk of developing localized cold injuries because there is decreased blood flow to the skin as the body attempts to further conserve fluids.

The most severe local cold injury is the result of tissue freezing and is referred to as *frostbite*. Much as is the case with a thermal burn, the depth of tissue injury depends on the length of time the tissue was exposed to the temperature extreme—the longer the exposure, the deeper and more severe the tissue injury. Early or superficial local cold injury results in a blanching, or pale discoloration, of the skin. On palpation of the affected area, it is noted that the firefighter has lost sensation in the area and that the skin remains pale without normal capillary refill on compression. Despite the color change, the skin remains soft to the touch. Some experts on environmental injuries have termed this early stage of tissue freezing as *frostnip*. If the affected area is rewarmed immediately, most patients at this early stage will have full recovery without permanent tissue loss. Patients will frequently complain of "tingling" sensations during rewarming tissue in these cases. This sensation usually is a symptom of the return of normal blood circulation to the area.

In late or deep freezing injury, the skin is pale white and "waxy" looking. On palpation, the skin will feel hard, like wood. Blisters and/or local swelling may also be seen. In severe cases of frostbite, as can be encountered with mountaineers, tissue as deep as muscle and bone may be frozen. As deep injuries begin to thaw, the affected skin may show a purple, blue, or mottled color.

Treatment of Local Cold Injuries   In general, the rewarming of local cold injury should take place in the controlled conditions of a hospital emergency department, not in the Rehab sector. The greatest risk associated with initiation of thawing an affected body part in the field is the possibility of its refreezing. Refreezing of partially thawed frostbitten areas drastically increases tissue injury and subsequent tissue loss. The goal of treatment of local cold injury is to prevent further injury or freezing of tissue.

Specific steps in the emergency care of localized cold injuries include:

1. Remove the firefighter from the cold environment.
2. Splint the affected extremity; do not allow the firefighter to walk on an affected extremity.
3. Cover the cold-injured area with dry clothing or dressings.

4. Remove any rings or jewelry from the affected area.
5. Do not rub or massage the area.
6. Do not break blisters.
7. Do not apply heat or attempt to rewarm the affected area.
8. Do not reexpose the area to a cold environment.

MEDICAL STAFFING OF THE REHAB SECTOR

The Rehab group/sector should be staffed with adequate personnel to provide medical evaluation and treatment and to assure that firefighters receive sufficient food and fluid replenishment. The most highly trained and qualified EMS personnel on the scene should provide medical evaluation and treatment in the Rehab group/sector. At the minimum, the area should be staffed by EMT-Bs. In large-scale incidents or in those where a trend toward serious heat- and stress-related illness is detected among firefighters, ALS units should be requested and assigned. At major incidents, some departments utilize an EMS-trained physician such as the department's medical director or fire surgeon in the rehab sector.

Often, outside EMS agencies such as mutual-aid companies or ambulance squads provide medical evaluation and treatment in the Rehab group/sector. If such agencies are used, it is essential that they have direct radio communication with Command.

Personnel without medical training can help provide food and fluid replenishment in the Rehab group/sector. In many volunteer fire departments, members of the department's Ladies' Auxiliary or an Explorer post fill this function. In addition, agencies such as the American Red Cross or local food retailers may offer additional nutritional support. When such organizations are involved in rehab, they must follow the directions of Command or the Rehab group/sector officer. This is especially important in order to assure that proper types of fluids—non-carbonated and caffeine-free—are administered.

Most of the space within the Rehab sector/group should be devoted to two large, clearly designated areas: the Rest and Refreshment area and the Medical Evaluation/Treatment area. Large tarps of different colors can be used to distinguish the two areas. Specifically assigning personnel who need assistance to these distinct areas makes monitoring and accountability during rehab easier.

MEDICAL EQUIPMENT IN THE REHAB SECTOR

It is essential that the rehab sector be stocked with appropriate and adequate medical supplies to attend the needs of firefighters. It is important to remember that providing medical care to emergency responders in rehab is a separate task from providing care to injured civilians at the same scene. Only in extraordinary circumstances should medical supplies or medical personnel in the Medical Evaluation/

Treatment Unit of rehab be tapped to provide non–rehab-related EMS care at the emergency scene.

Assembling and stocking of medical supplies for rehab should be based on treatment needs for the common types of illness and injuries incurred by firefighters on duty. However, provision should be made so that rehab personnel are prepared for catastrophic events such as sudden cardiac death.

One of the most common treatments in rehab is the administration of supplemental oxygen. A multiple-yoke oxygen system running from a large E cylinder is ideal for many rehab treatment areas, as it allows several firefighters to be treated from a single oxygen source. Small portable oxygen cylinders with regulators are also helpful when firefighters are more spread out, and are essential when firefighters who require oxygen are moved from the rehab area to an ambulance for transport to a hospital.

Basic EMS supplies should be routinely stocked in the treatment area of rehab. Additional supplies beyond those basic items are listed in Table 4-2. It is often helpful to prepackage all these supplies in large "rehab treatment boxes" to facilitate rapid and easy deployment of medical supplies to the rehab sector (Figure 4-5).

ENTRY AND TRIAGE

As noted, all crews must enter and exit the Rehab group/sector through a single designated entry point and be time-logged in by the sector staff. Upon entering rehab,

Table 4-2 Medical Supplies for Rehab*

Basic Life Support

Sterile burn and wound dressings
Liter containers of sterile saline solution for irrigation
Eye emergency kits
Oral or tympanic thermometers
Additional blood pressure cuffs for monitoring
Splints
Automated external defibrillator

Advanced Life Support

Defibrillator monitors
Additional liters of IV solution (normal saline)
Medications
   Full supply of ACLS drugs
   Opthalmic anesthetic
Morgan lens

*These supplies are in addition to standard EMS supplies such as jump kits, suction units, and portable oxygen cylinders.

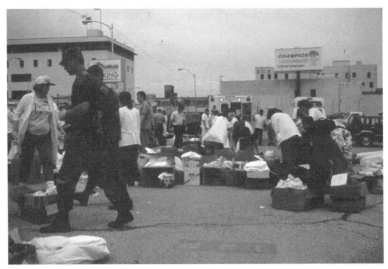

Figure 4-5 It is helpful to prepackage medical supplies for rehab in large boxes.

fire crews should be allowed to remove their SCBAs, hoods, and turnout gear. Once gear is removed, each crew member should be evaluated for injuries and for heat- and stress-related illnesses. The first step in evaluation is obtaining entry vital signs, including blood pressure and pulse. Rehab staff should rapidly question crew members, being alert to potentially life-threatening complaints such as the presence of chest pain or shortness of breath. Remember, the goal of the entry medical evaluation is to identify personnel with potential heat- or stress-related illnesses or injuries, not to keep firefighters from rest and rehydration.

When the entry evaluation is complete, rehab staff should assign crew members either to the Rest and Refreshment Unit or to the Medical Evaluation/ Treatment Unit. Firefighters assigned to the Medical Evaluation/Treatment Unit will receive more intensive evaluation and monitoring as well as rehydration and rest. The findings in the entry medical evaluation determine the area to which crew members are assigned. Local protocols vary, but firefighters who have a sustained pulse rate greater than 120 beats per minute at entry, who have markedly abnormal blood pressure, or who have sustained any injuries should be assigned to the Medical Evaluation/Treatment Unit (Table 4-3).

Table 4-3 Entry Evaluation Findings Mandating Triage to the Medical Evaluation/Treatment Unit

Heart rate	>120
Blood pressure	>200 systolic
	<90 systolic
	>110 diastolic
Injuries	Any

MEDICAL EVALUATION/TREATMENT UNIT

Crew members are triaged to the Medical Evaluation/Treatment Unit because their entry evaluations indicate a potential risk for having or developing heat- or stress-related illnesses. They may also be triaged to this area because of injuries they have sustained. Firefighters triaged with abnormal vital signs require ongoing assessment of their vital signs and conditions while they are resting and taking in oral rehydration and/or food. These firefighters should, at a minimum, have their vital signs reassessed 20 minutes after entering the Rehab group/sector. Each firefighter's sequential vital signs and assessments should be logged on a flow sheet (Figure 4-6). After 20 minutes of cooldown with rest and rehydration, the vital signs of most crew members will return to normal levels.

Some firefighters may still have elevated heart rates (greater than 100 beats per minute) after 20 minutes. These firefighters must generally remain in the Rehab group/sector for additional rehydration. Some jurisdictions have SOPs that prohibit such personnel from returning to duty for the remainder of the incident or shift.

The exact amount of time that crews should spend in the Rehab group/ sector will depend on their level of exhaustion and need for rest, rehydration, and—during prolonged operations—nutrition. At a minimum, crews should remain in the Rehab group/sector for 20 minutes of cool-down and rest time. Before returning to fire fighting or rescue duties, all crew members should have a repeat pulse and blood pressure check. If a crew member still has abnormal vital signs at this time, then the entire crew must remain in rehabilitation and receive additional rehabilitation and monitoring (Table 4-4).

All personnel who enter the Rehab group/sector with injuries should have those injuries promptly evaluated. Appropriate treatment should be given and transport to a medical facility provided if warranted. If a crew member is transported, other members of that crew can potentially go back on line. However, be sure that those crew members and Command are informed that a crew member has been

EMERGENCY INCIDENT REHABILITATION REPORT		INCIDENT: _Palmer Rd. structure fire_								
		DATE: _6/18/99_								

NAME / UNIT #	TIMES(S)	TIME /# Bottles	BP	PULSE	RESP	TEMP	SKIN	TAKEN BY	COMPLAINTS/CONDITION	TRANSPORT?
John Skoda	0940	NA	$140/70$	78	16	NA	NL	ETD	Swollen, deformed ankle	Yes/St. Mary's Hospital

Figure 4-6 The sequential vital signs of responders who have been sent to the Rehab group/sector should be logged on a flow sheet like this one.

Table 4-4 Reevaluation Findings Mandating Continued Time in the Rehab Group/Sector

Heart rate	>100
Blood pressure	>160 systolic
	<100 systolic
	>90 diastolic

transported and that appropriate adjustment has been made in the scene accountability system.

Because a goal of rehab operations is to detect and prevent heat-related emergencies, many fire department SOPs call for monitoring the firefighter's temperature. Some rehabilitation SOPs mandate obtaining oral or tympanic temperatures on all firefighters with heart rates greater than 110 to 120 beats per minute at entry into rehab. If the firefighter's temperature is greater than 100.6°F (38.1°C), then he or she is not permitted to put turnout gear or SCBA back on. For example, the Phoenix Fire Department's rehabilitation SOP states that any firefighter with a temperature higher than 101°F (38.3°C) must receive intravenous (IV) hydration and be transported to the emergency department.

In winter months, generalized hypothermia and local cold injuries such as frostbite must be considerations during medical evaluation of fire and rescue crews. In these conditions, the Rehab group/sector must provide crews with warmth and protection from ice and snow hazards. Remember, however, that heat- and stress-related illnesses, as well as dehydration, can also occur in cool and cold weather.

During rehabilitation and medical monitoring of crews, Rehab group/sector personnel may detect signs and symptoms of potentially life-threatening emergencies. These signs and symptoms include the following:

- Chest pain
- Shortness of breath
- Altered mental status (confusion, seizures, dizziness, etc.)
- Skin that is hot and either dry or moist
- Irregular pulse
- Oral temperature greater than 101°F (38.3°C).
- Pulse greater than 150 at any time
- Pulse greater than 140 after cooldown
- Systolic blood pressure greater than 200 mm Hg after cooldown
- Diastolic blood pressure greater than 130 mm Hg at any time

If any of these conditions is detected, place the firefighter on high-flow oxygen, initiate appropriate care, and transport the firefighter immediately to a hospital emergency department for further evaluation and treatment. Use of an ALS unit is indicated for all these conditions. However, transport from the Rehab group/sector should not be delayed if ALS is unavailable.

Whenever medical personnel assigned to the Rehab sector are unsure about the disposition of a firefighter who reports there, it is always better to act on the side of safety. Therefore, if your evaluation of a firefighter's condition indicates that he or she is marginal for return to active duty, keep that firefighter off duty. Similarly, if there is any question about whether a firefighter's signs or symptoms indicate a potentially dangerous condition, make sure that the firefighter is transported from Rehab to a medical facility for further evaluation and care.

One other thing that Rehab group/sector personnel must be on the look-out for when monitoring fire or rescue crews is a pattern of unusual complaints, illnesses, or injuries. Such patterns may indicate unexpected hazards involved in the incident. For example, if several firefighters at a fire scene complain of excessive salivation, runny noses, and diarrhea, it is a good indication that organophosphate pesticides are involved in the fire. Complaints of burning eyes could indicate the presence of metal gases. If unusual patterns such as these are noted, the EMT assigned to the Rehab group/sector must immediately report the finding to the Incident Commander so that appropriate actions can be taken.

Finally, firefighters and other rescue personnel who are initially sent to the Rest and Refreshment Unit in rehab but who are unable to tolerate oral rehydration due to nausea or vomiting should be reassigned or retriaged to the Medical Evaluation/Treatment Unit. These firefighters should be closely monitored. They will likely require IV hydration by ALS providers and will need to be transported to a hospital emergency department.

SUGGESTED READINGS

Dickinson, Edward T. *Fire Service Emergency Care.* Upper Saddle River, NJ: Brady–IFSTA, 1999.

FEMA–U.S. Fire Administration. *Emergency Incident Rehabilitation,* FA-114 July 1992. USFA Publications, P.O. Box 70274, Washington, DC 20024. Provides a sample EIR SOP.

5

FLUIDS AND NUTRITION IN REHAB

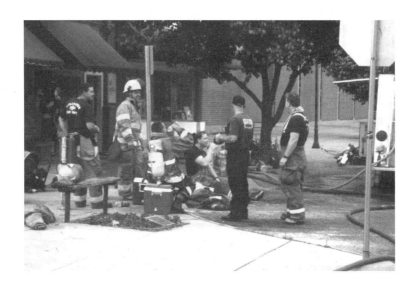

Long before the term *rehabilitation* was ever used in the fire service, a tradition existed of providing firefighters with food and beverages during prolonged fire scenes. The Ladies' Auxiliary who responded with coffee and doughnuts and the local restaurant owner who came in from home and turned the grill on for bacon-and-egg sandwiches at 3 A.M. are examples of this tradition. As well, parts of this tradition included less beneficial practices—such as a case of beer being brought from the local fire house and opened as soon as overhaul operations commenced.

Today, as a result of the creation of formal rehabilitation operations, there is an increased awareness of the need for proper replenishment for the fluid and nutritional losses incurred by firefighters during fire suppression and rescue operations. It is now recognized that replenishment of fluids is not simply a way of making firefighters "feel" better but is, in fact, a crucial component of maintaining overall well-being. Replenishing fluids can help in preventing dehydration, reducing the risk of certain heat-related emergencies, and lessening cardiovascular stress in already dehydrated firefighters.

BASIC CONCEPTS

The nutritional and fluid replenishment needs of firefighters will vary widely from one incident to another (Figure 5-1). While two coolers of a sports drink may be enough for an engine company working at a single room and contents fire, it will certainly not suffice for a crew of firefighters involved in wildland fire suppression for 16 hours. Similarly, it may be easy to provide hot soup and grilled ham-and-cheese sandwiches to firefighters at a prolonged suburban mall fire but impractical to cook such meals during a high-angle rescue operation in the remote back country.

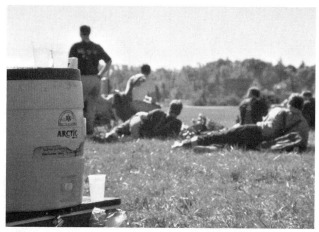

Figure 5-1   Supplying beverages for fluid replenishment is a key task for workers in the Rehab group/sector.

In general practice, the components to be considered in providing nutritional support in rehab can be thought of as a triangle (Figure 5-2). The triangle's sides are made up of (1) the fluid/nutritional needs of the personnel, (2) the local resources available to provide for these needs, and (3) the ability of firefighters to retain and digest the fluids or food provided. By balancing these three factors, the appropriate type of fluid—and, perhaps, food—replenishment can be determined for the personnel at a given incident.

The ability of local resources to provide the necessary fluid and nutritional support will be affected by a variety of considerations such as the remoteness of the emergency scene and the availability of refrigeration. The nutritional needs of the firefighters and their ability to digest the fluids and foods provided are based on nutritional science and physiology.

In all circumstances, the Rehab group/sector must provide adequate water, electrolytes, and energy-producing carbohydrates to assure that firefighters and other rescue personnel can continue to function safely and at optimal levels, despite adverse environmental and physiological conditions.

FLUIDS AND ELECTROLYTES

In the vast majority of operations, the personnel staffing rehab will only have to supply fluids rather than solid foods too. Therefore, an understanding of the functions of fluids and electrolytes and of the key concept of maintaining *water balance* is essential to effective rehab operations.

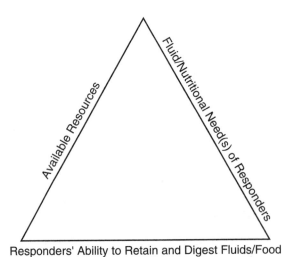

Figure 5-2   Components of nutritional support in rehab.

Water and Water Balance

Approximately 60 percent of the body's total weight is comprised of water. All the cells in the body contain some amount of water, and some cells hold a higher proportion than others. For example, muscle cells have a higher water content than fat cells. This means that a well-toned, muscular firefighter will have higher fluid requirements than a firefighter who weighs the same amount but whose body has a greater percentage of fat. The term *hydration* refers to the amount of water the body contains. In normal baseline conditions, the body is adequately hydrated. This means there is a proper fluid balance between the water lost by the body in its normal functioning and the oral intake of fluids in the form of liquids and foods that contain water.

The body loses water by several routes. For example, fluids are lost in urine, in stool, in exhalation, and in sweat. At normal levels of activity (sitting around the firehouse reading a magazine), most water is lost through urination. When the body is in a hot environment or engaged in prolonged or intense physical activity (advancing a $1^3/_4$-inch hose line down a fire-filled hall), the largest water loss is through sweating, as the body works to maintain a constant temperature by cooling itself through the evaporation of perspiration.

The actual volume of fluid lost to sweating during strenuous physical activity will vary with an individual's metabolism, the degree of activity, and the environmental temperature. Sweat losses of about 1 liter per hour are common, however.

Loss of adequate hydration, or *dehydration,* is inevitable with increased fluid loss during prolonged exposure to heat or strenuous activity unless water is returned to the body by oral intake. If dehydration is allowed to progress without adequate *rehydration,* or replenishment of water, firefighter performance will begin to be affected (Figure 5-3). Indeed, if just 4 percent of body weight is lost in water from sweating (not an unrealistic possibility in extended operations such as wildland fire suppression), both mental and physical abilities may be compromised. (It should be mentioned that *overhydration* can sometimes occur. This situation, in which fluids are ingested far in excess of the amounts lost, will be discussed later in the chapter.)

Dehydration has the potential to pose additional risks to fire and rescue personnel because of the relationship between dehydration and the body's ability to regulate its core temperature (thermoregulation). As the body becomes progressively more dehydrated, core temperature begins to rise. This means that dehydrated firefighters are placed at even greater risk for heat-related emergencies, in addition to those such as heat cramps that are caused by loss of electrolytes in the sweat (see Chapter 4).

In situations where dehydration begins to develop, the body itself takes steps to retain as much water as possible while still having to lose water in the form of sweat. The kidneys and parts of the adrenal glands are extremely sensitive to water balance. In situations of developing dehydration, the kidneys will reduce both the amount of urine produced and the amount of water contained in the urine. Thus, firefighters experiencing dehydration, or so-called "negative water balance,"

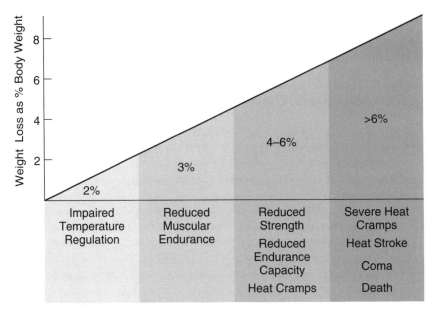

Figure 5-3   The effects of dehydration on body functions.

will note less frequent urination and darker, stronger-smelling urine as the kidneys work to retain water.

In extended operations, firefighters should be trained to monitor themselves for signs of dehydration. The most obvious of these signs is, of course, thirst, but this is often an unreliable marker of true dehydration. Firefighters should also be trained to monitor the frequency, quantity, and characteristics of their urination as key indicators of water balance. Normal urine from a well-hydrated individual should be almost clear in color and without much odor. Urine that is dark or deep yellow in color and has a strong odor is an indication that a negative water balance has developed and that the firefighter needs immediate rehydration (see section on rehydration). It should be noted that certain types of foods and vitamins may alter the color and smell of urine. Vitamin B compounds taken as dietary supplements will give urine a bright yellow color and a characteristic smell. In addition, foods containing asparagus will cause most individuals to develop a foul "swamp water" smell to their urine.

Assuring that the body maintains a balance between water lost and water replaced is essential to a firefighter's well-being. A key function of rehab operations is to provide the opportunity and resources to maintain this balance. Failing to maintain a proper water balance and allowing dehydration to develop may have significant, even catastrophic, consequences.

Electrolytes

Just as water balance is an essential component of body physiology, so too is electrolyte balance. *Electrolytes* are chemically charged elements essential to proper cell function in virtually all organ systems. Key electrolytes include sodium, potassium, calcium, and magnesium. The electrolytes acting on cells and cell membranes allow for a wide variety of cell activities including the movement of skeletal muscle and the beating of the heart. Marked shifts in the amounts of electrolytes in the body can result in dysfunction of much of the body's normal physiology.

The two following examples illustrate the importance of proper electrolyte balance. If levels of sodium fall too low, which can occur with excessive sweating, a loss of proper skeletal muscle functioning can result. Clinically, this loss of proper muscle functioning leads to heat cramps, which are common in hot environments when excessive sodium is lost in sweat but not adequately replaced by oral intake. Similarly, the presence of excessively high or excessively low levels of potassium in the blood can result in cardiac arrest because the heart's electrical system loses its ability to properly generate and conduct electrical impulses. This disruption of electrical activity in the heart can cause potentially lethal cardiac arrhythmias, including ventricular tachycardia and ventricular fibrillation.

Electrolytes are lost from the body by the same mechanisms through which water is lost from the body. As with water, most electrolytes are lost in the form of sweat and urine, sweat being the primary mechanism of loss during periods of strenuous activity. The characteristic salty taste of sweat is due to its high sodium content.

The kidneys and adrenal glands again play crucial roles in the body's effort to retain electrolytes in compensation for loss through sweating. The kidneys will avidly retain sodium when the body senses that sodium is becoming depleted. Firefighters who may be taking a class of drugs called diuretics, or "water pills," such as Lasix (furosemide) will lose excessive amounts of electrolytes, especially potassium and magnesium, because of their prescription medication. These firefighters are at particular risk for electrolyte abnormalities.

During prolonged exertion, it will be necessary to replenish both water and electrolytes as part of rehydration.

Carbohydrates

Water and electrolytes provide the body with essential elements that help assure normal cell and organ function. Neither water nor electrolytes, however, provide the body with molecules that are capable of producing energy within the body. It is *carbohydrates* that are the chemical substances responsible for producing the energy that drives body metabolism.

Carbohydrates are molecules made up of carbon (C), hydrogen (H), and oxygen (O) atoms. They exist in two basic forms, simple carbohydrates and complex carbohydrates. Examples of simple carbohydrates include sugars such as glucose, sucrose, dextrose, lactose, and fructose. These sugars are readily available sources of energy and can be found in a variety of natural foods (Table 5-1).

Complex carbohydrates are defined as molecules made up of three or more sugars. The main sources of complex carbohydrates are starches such as bread, pasta, and potatoes.

Once complex carbohydrates are ingested, they are converted to simple sugars (usually glucose), which are then used by the brain, muscles, and other organs as essential sources of energy. The body cannot function without adequate glucose. Lack of glucose leads to cellular dysfunction. An example of a medical emergency that involves a lack of glucose is hypoglycemia, or "insulin shock." This condition often occurs in insulin-dependent diabetic patients. These patients experience altered mental status, confusion, and even unresponsiveness because of the lack of adequate glucose.

During physical activity, the body increases its use of carbohydrates in order to allow it to function at optimal performance levels. This "burning" of carbohydrates by cells depletes the body's carbohydrate stores much like sweating and urination deplete its water and electrolyte stores. The body has only a very limited ability to store carbohydrates. Only glycogen can be stored in limited quantities in the body's muscle and liver tissues.

Because of the body's limited ability to store carbohydrates, carbohydrates must also be provided to emergency responders sent to rehab as part of fluid and food replenishment. Because it takes time for the body to convert complex carbohydrates into usable forms of simple sugars, it is preferable that first-line carbohydrate replenishment be in the form of simple carbohydrates. This makes energy more immediately available to the body's cells. This is why most commercially available sports drinks contain simple carbohydrates as well as water and electrolytes. In prolonged operations where food will be provided, complex carbohydrates can be provided in the form of starchy foods such as pastas and stews.

Replenishment Strategies

Assuring that the body maintains adequate amounts of water, electrolytes, and carbohydrates to permit proper functioning of the body's cells and organs is essential

Table 5-1   Sources of Simple Carbohydrates

Type of Sugar	Food Source
Sucrose	Table sugar
Fructose and glucose	Honey
Fructose	Fruit
Lactose	Milk

to a firefighter's well-being. This goal can be obtained by two basic strategies, pre-hydration and rehydration.

Prehydration

The concept of *prehydration* is based upon assuring that a firefighter is adequately hydrated at all times and, if possible, enters into an emergency scene with a slightly positive water balance. Strategies for maintaining adequate hydration include the following:

- Avoiding excessive use of caffeinated beverages while on duty, as these liquids promote excessive urination.
- Avoiding excessive alcohol use before coming on duty; residual dehydration is common with hangovers.
- Being aggressive about personal rehydration after strenuous, non–duty-related activities such as competitive sports or running.
- Monitoring urine, which is a sensitive indicator of hydration status. Urine should be clear in color and odor free. Increase fluid intake if urine darkens.

With the exception of certain prolonged operations, it will be difficult to be able to predict exactly when a major response will occur that will place the firefighter in extreme physiological stress. If it is known that a physiologically stressful event is inevitable within an hour or two—for example, with a task force moving up from staging—then prehydration to create a positive water balance should be initiated. The U.S. Navy SEALs recommend prehydration strategies based on the type and duration of anticipated activity (Table 5-2).

Some fire departments in the Southwest require their firefighters to maintain prehydration status while on duty during periods of prolonged high temperatures. Such policies often require on-duty personnel to drink 6 to 8 ounces of fluid every 6 hours while on duty in addition to intake of their regular meals. Obviously, such routine prehydration strategies may be difficult to accomplish for volunteer firefighters.

Be aware that overly aggressive prehydration can lead to overhydration. Overhydration is especially detrimental when plain water is used, because key electrolytes such as sodium and potassium can be diluted out when too much water is taken in. In a hot environment especially, a firefighter who starts out with low

Table 5-2 Prehydration Strategies

Intensity of Activity	Duration	Fluid Recommendation*
High	Less than 1 hour	8 to 16 ounces of carbohydrate-containing fluid, 1 or 2 hours before the operation
Moderate to high	1 to 3 hours	8 to 16 ounces of water per hour, 0 to 2 hours before the operation

*During periods of extreme heat, it may be necessary to double these recommendations.

electrolyte levels risks more rapid development of electrolyte-mediated heat emergencies such as heat cramps and heat exhaustion. To avoid such risks, electrolytes and carbohydrates—as well as water—should be part of the makeup of hydration fluids.

Rehydration

Rehydration is the principal nutritional function of the rehab sector. Firefighters who enter rehab should begin rehydration as soon as baseline vital signs are taken and accountability requirements have been met.

Although there may be some local variations, ideal rehydration solutions administered in rehab operations should, as noted, contain not only water but electrolytes and simple carbohydrates as well. Commercial sports drinks are readily obtainable beverages that contain these three major components. Examples of commonly available sports drinks and their contents are listed in Table 5-3.

There are two additional considerations when choosing a liquid for use in rehab. First, the beverage must have a taste acceptable to the firefighters who will be consuming it. Although taste is a matter of individual preference, the simple sugars contained in most commercially available rehydration solutions make these drinks palatable to large numbers of users.

Table 5-3 Characteristics of Beverages Commonly Used for Rehydration

Beverage*	Types of Sugars and Concentration	Sodium, mg	Potassium, mg	Other Nutrients	Osmolarity, mOsm/L
Gatorade	6% sucrose/glucose	110	25	Chloride, phosphorus	280–360
Exceed	7.2% glucose polymers/ fructose	50	45	Chloride, calcium, magnesium, phosphorus	250
Body Fuel	4.2% maltodextrin/fructose	80	20	Phosphorus, chloride, iron, vitamins A, B, C	210
10-K	6.3% sucrose/glucose/ fructose	52	26	Phosphorus, vitamin C, chloride	350
Quickick	4.7% fructose/sucrose	116	23	Calcium, chloride, phosphorus	305
Coca-Cola	11% high-fructose corn syrup/sucrose	9.2	Trace	Phosphorus	600–715
Sprite	10.2% high-fructose corn syrup/sucrose	28	Trace	...	695
Cranberry Juice Cocktail	15% high-fructose corn syrup/sucrose	10	61	Vitamin C, phosphorus	890
Orange juice	11.8% fructose/sucrose/ glucose	2.7	510	Calcium, niacin, iron, vitamins A and C, thiamine, phosphorus, riboflavin	690
Water	...	Low	Low	Low	10–20

*Serving size: 8 fluid ounces.
Source: *The Navy SEAL Nutrition Guide.*

The second consideration is that the beverage must be easily tolerated by the gastrointestinal (GI) system. It must not cause nausea, vomiting, or other adverse effects.

Several factors affect how well rehydration solutions are tolerated by the GI system. The first of these is temperature. Rehydration fluids should generally never be served at the extremes of temperature. When rehydrating in hot conditions, fluids should be cool but not ice cold. Rapid ingestion of ice-cold fluids can cause painful spasms of the esophagus or even—rarely—precipitous slowing of the heart rate. Similarly, in cold conditions, "hot" rehydration beverages should be served warm rather than piping hot.

Another factor that contributes to the digestion of a fluid is its *osmolarity*. Osmolarity can be roughly defined as the "thickness" of a fluid as determined by the electrolyte and carbohydrate content of the beverage. The higher the osmolarity, the longer the time it will take to absorb the fluid and the harder the fluid will be to digest. In general, it is recommended that rehydration solutions served in rehab do not exceed an osmolarity of 350 mOsm/liter.

The osmolarities of various widely used rehydration solutions are listed in Table 5-3. If a commercially available beverage exceeds the recommended limit of 350 mOsm/liter, the beverage can simply be diluted with water in order to comply with this guideline.

The final factor in GI tolerance is prevention of stomach or gastric distention. Gastric distention can result in such unpleasantness as abdominal pain, "heartburn"/reflux, or even vomiting. Gastric distention can be minimized by taking the following steps:

- Assuring that the rehydration solutions have an osmolarity less than 350 mOsm/liter
- Assuring that rehydration solutions are administered in reasonable rather than excessive amounts
- Assuring that rehydration solutions are not carbonated

The rate at which the stomach is able to empty its contents into the intestine (gastric emptying rate) also has a major impact on GI tolerance of oral fluid replacement. Gastric emptying rates in adult males of average weight are about 1.0 to 1.5 liters per hour. The gastric emptying rate, however, can be reduced by several factors that directly impact firefighters involved in rescue and fire suppression activities. These factors include high-intensity activity, heat stress, and dehydration itself. Therefore, firefighters who are hot, exhausted, and dehydrated from strenuous activity may be less able to tolerate larger volumes of rehydration solutions and be at greater risk of developing complications of gastric distention (including nausea and vomiting).

Once an appropriate rehydration solution is selected, it should be administered to all firefighters in the Rehab group/sector except for those who are highly nauseated or those who are vomiting (these personnel will require IV rehydration).

Fluid replenishment should be provided throughout emergency scene operations as crews rotate through rehab. Rehydration should *also* be provided when personnel are released from active on-scene duties and are back in quarters.

As a rule of thumb, crews rotating through rehab who are recovering from high-intensity physical activity should receive between 12 and 32 ounces of rehydration fluids during a 30-minute rotation in rehabilitation. Note that this figure is only a benchmark; the amount of fluid provided will depend upon the level of dehydration. After operations are completed, firefighters should ingest an additional 8 to 32 ounces of electrolyte- and carbohydrate-containing fluids over the 2 hours following the operation. Firefighters should monitor their urine after the completion of an operation. If a firefighter notes that his or her urine continues to be dark in color or strong in odor after returning to the station or home, then additional rehydration will be necessary to restore a proper water balance.

PROVISION OF SOLID FOODS IN REHAB

In prolonged operations such as wildland fire suppression or urban search and rescue operations, firefighters and other emergency personnel must receive not only adequate fluid rehydration but also more comprehensive nutritional support in the form of solid foods and meals.

The provision of this solid food in these circumstances is less well understood and studied than is fluid rehydration. Often, when replenishment operations move into the realm of solid foods, they are handed over to outside vendors and agencies such as the Red Cross, which then provide nutritional support. No matter who is responsible for providing them, the solid foods served to firefighters must meet two basic criteria—they must supply adequate and carefully thought-out nutrition, and they must be able to be served easily and safely to emergency personnel on the scene.

To understand more about the types of foods to serve at rehab operations, an understanding of some basics of nutrition is necessary. Consider first the three major types of nutrients that make up a normal diet. These include carbohydrates, fats, and proteins.

Carbohydrates

Carbohydrates, as noted above, are the primary source of energy in human metabolism, providing glucose for energy. Glucose is essential for proper functioning of many organ systems in the body. Most importantly for firefighters, glucose is essential for optimal performance of skeletal muscles and the brain. In an earlier section on rehydration, discussion focused on the simple carbohydrates or sugars contained in rehydration solutions. When dealing with solid foods, both simple and complex carbohydrates are commonly encountered. Complex carbohydrates provide a more sustained source of energy because they are converted more slowly to "usable" simple carbohydrates through the process of digestion in the gastrointestinal tract.

The conversion of complex carbohydrates to sugars begins in the mouth as chemicals contained in saliva initiate the process of digestion. This first step in carbohydrate digestion accounts for the fact that bread begins to taste progressively sweeter in the mouth the longer it is chewed and exposed to saliva. Common foods that contain complex carbohydrates include breads, pastas, rice, potatoes, and other starchy foods.

Because of their crucial energy-producing role in body metabolism, carbohydrates should be the most prevalent nutrient group contained in foods supplied to firefighters and rescue personnel in rehab during prolonged operations.

Fats

Fats represent another source of energy for the body. While the body provides only limited storage for carbohydrates in the form of glycogen, fat can be readily stored. Fat is a particularly important source of energy during prolonged exercise, in cold environments, and in extreme conditions where carbohydrates are no longer available to provide energy for metabolism. For these reasons, fat-free foods are not necessarily to be sought out for rehab operations. Fat, in moderation, should certainly be included in the foods provided in rehab.

Proteins

Proteins are nitrogen-containing compounds that have importance for a wide variety of crucial structures and functions within the body. These functions include:

- Service as chemical messengers in the body facilitating the transport of fats and other nutrients throughout the body
- Provision of some energy to the body
- Formation of muscles and other key body structures
- Repair of injuries to body tissues

Proteins are made up of smaller molecules of amino acids. The body can synthesize many amino acids. However, nine amino acids (so-called essential amino acids) can only be obtained through dietary intake. The body requires only relatively small amounts of essential amino acids in the diet, but a lack of these acids will result in loss of proteins needed for normal body structure, repair, and function.

Although proteins are only a minor source of energy production in the body, their various other functions mean that proteins are essential components of foods chosen for rehab operations. Routine sources of dietary proteins are meats, fish, and milk products including cheese.

Determining Specific Foods for Rehab

As stated previously, whatever food is selected for the rehab sector, it must be locally available and practically "servable" at the emergency incident scene. Logistical considerations such as being able to prepare, store, and serve the food in sanitary conditions will help determine what foods to select. For example, bologna-and-cheese sandwiches served with cups of a hearty stew may be ideal choices from a nutritional aspect. However, if the sandwiches spoil because of a lack of refrigeration or the stew cannot be served warm because there are no stoves, then the choice is impractical. Even worse, the serving of improperly stored or prepared food raises the risk of food-borne bacteria such as staph., *E. coli* or salmonella incapacitating all personnel at an emergency scene with vomiting and diarrhea.

Every department's SOPs for major incidents should include preplanned menus indicating exactly what types of foods will be served in rehab during prolonged operations. These menus should be based on sound nutritional considerations as well as on realistic considerations of the requirements of food preparation, storage, and delivery on the scene.

Minor Nutritional Support

At some medium-duration incidents, it may only be necessary to provide personnel with snack-type foods. With these incidents, complex carbohydrates are perhaps the most important component of any solid foods provided to on-scene personnel. Fruits such as oranges, bananas, and apples are excellent sources of complex carbohydrates; they possess the added benefit of having high water content to supplement oral rehydration with liquids. In addition, fruit is easily stored and served in virtually any rehabilitation setting.

Some departments use commercially available, individually packaged snack bars for minor nutritional support. There are over 50 types of such bars on the market currently. Most of these bars are reasonable sources of necessary carbohydrates, fat, and protein. Table 5-4 shows samples of the nutritional content of several commercial snack bars. A common complaint with these snack, sports, or "energy" bars is that some taste like "sawdust"—or worse. It is an excellent idea to have department members taste-test these bars prior to use in rehab and reach a consensus on an acceptable brand. It does little good to rely on such bars for necessary minor nutritional support when no one is willing to eat them.

Note that the wrappers of individually packaged foods can produce a considerable amount of trash. Remember to provide trash receptacles in the Rehab group/sector.

Table 5-4   Nutritional Content of Assorted Commercial Snack Bars

	Nature Valley	Golf Pro	Breakthru	Tiger's Milk	Nutri-Grain	Power Bar
Carbohydrates, grams	28–29	35–40	37–39	18–24	27	45
Fat, grams	6	3–6	3	2.5–6	3	2–2.5
Protein, grams	4–5	4.5–10	10–12	4–7	2	10
Calories	180–190	205–235	220–230	130–150	140	230

Source: *Golf Digest*, October 1998.

Major Nutritional Support

In prolonged operations, it may be necessary to provide responders with more "meal"-like foods as part of rehab operations. Providing meals for a large ongoing operation can represent a huge drain on departmental resources that are likely to have already been spread thin because of the magnitude of the emergency incident. For this reason, the assistance of outside agencies and organizations like the American Red Cross, fire buff organizations, or departmental Ladies' Auxiliaries is most helpful when major nutritional support is required (Figure 5-4). Some larger fire departments do have the capability of providing major nutritional support services at extended incidents, but they are exceptions.

Departments should sit down with the organization(s) that will provide major nutritional support and study the logistics of the job. The plan that results from this discussion should become a component of departmental SOPs for rehab operations at extended incidents. Elements that should be considered when planning nutritional support operations with outside organizations include the following:

- Menu planning based on local resources and sound nutrition
- Staffing requirements
- Procedures for notification or request for aid from the organization(s)
- Orientation of the outside organization(s) to the Incident Command System
- Legal considerations including contractual obligations and appropriate liability insurance

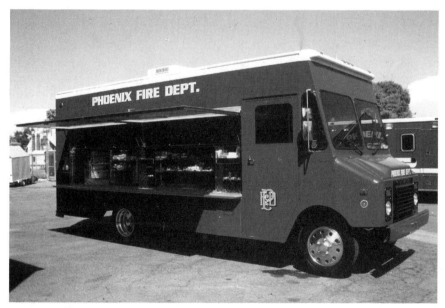

Figure 5-4a   Some fire departments have their own resources for major nutritional support (A), while other departments make arrangements with outside agencies and organizations (B).

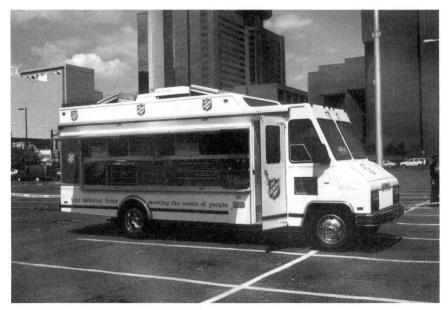

Figure 5-4b

CONCLUSION

Provision of fluid and nutritional support to firefighters is a key part of rehab operations. Departmental SOPs should have clearly specified guidelines for the preparation, storage, and serving of both liquids for rehydration and food for minor and major nutritional support. Remember—a pumper will function with the amount of water it brings with it in its booster tank to the fire scene for only a limited time before it runs out and needs to be resupplied. In the same way, the bodies of firefighters will work efficiently for only a limited time on the fluid and nutritional resources they bring within them to the fire scene before needing replenishment in the Rehab group/sector.

SUGGESTED READINGS

Deuster, Patricia A., et al. *The Navy SEAL Nutrition Guide.* Bethesda, MD: Dept. of Military and Emergency Medicine of the Uniformed Sources, University of Health Sciences, F. Edward Hubert School of Medicine (1994).

Sawka, M. N. "Physiological consequences of hypohydration: Exercise performance and thermoregulation," *Medicine and Science in Sports and Exercise, 24*(6): 657–669, 1992.

INDEX